Histological Typing of Prostate Tumours

Springer-Verlag Berlin Heidelberg GmbH

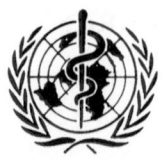 World Health Organization

The series *International Histological Classification of Tumours* consists of the following volumes. The early ones can be ordered through WHO, Distribution and Sales, Avenue Appia, CH-1211 Geneva 27.

2. Histological typing of breast tumours (1968, second edition 1981)
14. Histological and cytological typing of neoplastic diseases of haematopoietic and lymphoid tissues (1976)

A coded compendium of the International Histological Classification of Tumours (1978).

The following volumes have already appeared in a revised second edition with Springer-Verlag:
Histological Typing of Thyroid Tumours. Hedinger/Williams/Sobin (1988)
Histological Typing of Intestinal Tumours. Jass/Sobin (1989)
Histological Typing of Oesophageal and Gastric Tumours. Watanabe/Jass/Sobin (1990)
Histological Typing of Tumours of the Gallbladder and Extrahepatic Bile Ducts. Albores-Saavedra/Henson/Sobin (1990)
Histological Typing of Tumours of the Upper Respiratory Tract and Ear. Shanmugaratnam/Sobin (1981)
Histological Typing of Salivary Gland Tumours. Seifert (1991)
Histological Typing of Odontogenic Tumours. Kramer/Pindborg/Shear (1992)
Histological Typing of Tumours of the Central Nervous System. Kleihues/Burger/Scheithauer (1993)
Histological Typing of Bone Tumours. Schajowicz (1993)
Histological Typing of Soft Tissue Tumours. Weiss (1994)
Histological Typing of Female Genital Tract Tumours. Scully et al. (1994)
Histological Typing of Tumours of the Liver. Ishak et al. (1994)
Histological Typing of Tumours of the Exocrine Pancreas. Klöppel/Solcia/Longnecker/Capella/Sobin (1996)
Histological Typing of Skin Tumours. Heenan/Elder/Sobin (1996)
Histological Typing of Cancer and Precancer of the Oral Mucosa. Pindborg/Reichart/Smith/van der Waal (1997)
Histological Typing of Kidney Tumours. Mostofi/Davis (1998)
Histological Typing of Testis Tumours. Mostofi/Sesterhenn (1998)
Histological Typing of Tumours of the Eye and Its Adnexa. Campbell (1998)
Histological Typing of Ovarian Tumours. Scully (1999)
Histological Typing of Lung and Pleural Tumours. Travis/Colby/Corrin (1999 third edition)
Histological Typing of Urinary Bladder Tumours. Mostofi/Davis/Sesterhenn (1999)
Histological Typing of Tumours of the Thymus. Rosai (1999)
Histological Typing of Endocrine Tumours. Solcia/Klöppel/Sobin (2000)
Histological Typing of Prostate Tumours. Mostofi/Sesterhenn/Davis (2002)

Histological Typing of Prostate Tumours

F.K. Mostofi I.A. Sesterhenn C.J. Davis, Jr.

In Collaboration with L.H. Sobin
and Participants from 10 Countries

Second Edition

With 146 Colour Figures

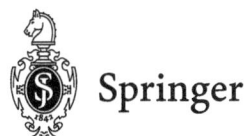 Springer

F.K. Mostofi, MD
I.A. Sesterhenn, MD
C.J. Davis, Jr., MD

WHO Collaborating Center for Histological Classification
of Tumours of Urinary Tract and Male Genital System
Armed Forces Institute of Pathology
Washington, DC 20306-6000, USA

L.H. Sobin, MD
WHO Collaborating Center for the International Histological
Classification of Tumours, Armed Forces Institute of Pathology
Washington, DC 20306-6000, USA

First edition published by WHO in 1980 as No. 22 in the International Histological
Classification of Tumours series.

ISBN 978-3-540-42256-3

Library of Congress Cataloging-in-Publication Data
Mostofi, F.K. (Fathollah Keshvar), 1911- Histological typing of prostate tumours/F.K. Mostofi, I.A.
Sesterhenn, C.J. Davis; in collaboration with L.H. Sobin and participants from 10 countries. - 2nd ed.
p. cm. - (International histological classification of tumours) Includes bibliographical references and
index.
ISBN 978-3-540-42256-3   ISBN 978-3-662-04888-7 (eBook)
DOI 10.1007/978-3-662-04888-7
1. Prostate-Tumors-Histopathology. 2. Prostate-Tumors-Classification. 3. Prostate-Tumors-Atlases.
I. Sesterhenn, I. II. Davis, Charles J. III. Sobin, L.H. IV. Title. V. International histological classification of tumours (Unnumbered)   RC280.P7 M675   2002   616.99'463-dc21   2001049437

http://www.springer.de

© Springer-Verlag Berlin Heidelberg 2002
Originally published by Springer-Verlag Berlin Heidelberg New York in 2002

Typesetting: Data conversion by Springer-Verlag, Heidelberg

Printed on acid-free paper.   SPIN 10833853   24/3130 ih – 5 4 3 2 1 0

Participants

Algaba F.
Department of Pathology, Fundacion Puigvert, Barcelona, Spain

Andersson L.
WHO Collaborating Center for Urologic Tumours,
Department of Urology, Karolinska Hospital, Stockholm, Sweden

Billis A.
Department of Anatomic Pathology, University Hospital,
School of Medicine, State University of Campinas (UNICAMP),
Campinas, Brazil

Carbillet J.P.
Department of Pathology, Service d'Anatomie et Cytologie
Pathologiques, Centre Hospitalier et Universitaire Besançon,
Besançon, France

Chan C.W.
Department of Anatomic and Cellular Pathology.
The Chinese University of Hong Kong, Hong Kong, China

Davis C.J., Jr.
Department of Genitourinary Pathology, Armed Forces Institute
of Pathology, Washington, DC, USA

Foster C.S.
Department of Pathology, Royal Liverpool University Hospital,
Liverpool, UK

Furusato M.
Department of Pathology, Kyorin University, Tokyo, Japan

Helpap B.
Department of Pathology, Hegan-Klinikum, Singen, Germany

Mostofi F.K.
Department of Genitourinary Pathology, Armed Forces Institute
of Pathology, Washington, DC, USA

Olchovskaya I.
Department of Pathology, Cancer Research Centre of the Russian
Academy of Medical Sciences, Moscow, Russia

Sesterhenn I.A.
Department of Genitourinary Pathology, Armed Forces Institute
of Pathology, Washington, DC, USA

Tribukait B.
Department of Medical Radiology, Karolinska Institute, Stockholm,
Sweden

General Preface to the Series

Among the prerequisites for comparative studies of cancer are international agreement on histological criteria for the classification of cancer types and a standardised nomenclature. At present, pathologists use different terms for the same pathological entity and, furthermore, the same term is sometimes applied to lesions of different types. An internationally agreed classification of tumours, acceptable alike to physicians, surgeons, radiologists, pathologists, and statisticians, would enable workers in all parts of the world to compare their findings and facilitate collaboration.

In a report published in 1952[1] a subcommittee of the WHO Expert Committee on Health Statistics discussed the general principles that should govern the statistical classification of tumours and agreed that, to ensure the necessary flexibility and ease in coding, three separate classifications were needed according to (1) anatomical site, (2) histological type, and (3) degree of malignancy. A classification according to anatomical site is available in the International Classification of Diseases[2].

In 1956, the WHO Executive Board passed a resolution[3] requesting the Director General to explore the possibility that the WHO might organise centres in various parts of the world and arrange for the collection of human tissues and their histological classification.

The main purpose of such centres would be to develop histological definitions of cancer types and to facilitate the wide adoption of a uniform nomenclature. This resolution was endorsed by the Tenth World Health Assembly in May 1957[4].

---

[1] WHO (1952) WHO Technical Report Series, no. 53. WHO, Geneva, p. 45.

[2] WHO (1977) Manual of the international statistical classification of diseases, injuries, and causes of death, 1975 version. WHO, Geneva.

[3] WHO (1956) WHO Official Records, no. 68, p. 14 (Resolution EB 17.R40).

[4] WHO (1957) WHO Official Records, no. 79, p. 467 (Resolution WHA 10.18).

Since 1958, the WHO has established a number of centres concerned with this subject. The result of this endeavour has been the International Histological Classification of Tumours, a multivolume series. The first edition was published between 1967 and 1981. The present, revised second edition aims to update the classification, reflecting progress in diagnoses and relevance of tumour types to clinical and epidemiologic features.

Preface to Histological Typing of Prostate Tumours – Second Edition

The first edition of the *International Histological Classification of Prostate Tumours* was published in 1981[1]. Since then, a number of new entities have been recognised, necessitating revision of the classification.

It will be appreciated, of course, that the classification reflects the existing state of knowledge, and modifications are certain to be needed as experience accumulates. Although the present classification has been adopted and recommended by the members of the group, it represents a view from which some pathologists may wish to dissent. It is hoped that, in the interests of international cooperation, all pathologists will try to use the classification as proposed. Criticisms and suggestions for its improvement are welcome. These should be sent to the World Health Organization, 1211 Geneva 27, Switzerland.

The histological classification which appears on pages 12–15 contains the corresponding morphology code numbers for tumours of the *International Classification of Diseases for Oncology* (ICD-O)[2] and of the *Systematized Nomenclature of Medicine* (SNOMED)[3].

The publications in the series *International Histological Classification of Tumours* are not intended to serve as textbooks but rather to promote the adoption of a uniform terminology of tumours that will facilitate and improve communication among cancer workers. For this reason, we have cited only two literature references. Readers should, therefore, refer to standard works on the subject for bibliographies.

---

[1] Mostofi FK, Sesterhenn IA, Sobin LH (1980) Histologic typing of prostate tumours. World Health Organization, Geneva (International Histological Classification of Tumours, No. 22).

[2] World Health Organization (2000) International Classification of Diseases for Oncology (ICD-O), third edn. Geneva.

[3] College of American Pathologists (http://snomed.org).

Contents

Introduction

This classification is based primarily on the microscopic characteristics of tumours and therefore is concerned with morphologically identifiable cell types and histological patterns as seen with conventional light microscopy.

The term *tumour* is used synonymously with *neoplasm*. The phrase *tumour-like* is applied to lesions that clinically or morphologically resemble neoplasms but do not behave biologically in a neoplastic manner. They are included in this publication because they give rise to problems in differential diagnosis and because of the unclear distinction between neoplasms and certain non-neoplastic lesions. Synonyms are listed only if they have been widely used or are considered helpful for the understanding of the lesion. In such cases, the preferred term is given first and followed by the synonym.

The current revision includes the recognition of a preinvasive lesion, prostatic intraepithelial neoplasia, which is commonly associated with carcinoma. It also recognises the paracrine-endocrine elements in prostate carcinoma and other subtypes of adenocarcinoma.

Although the emphasis of the classification is on histological typing, consideration should also be given to the degree of differentiation and nuclear anaplasia, extent of local spread, vascular and lymphatic invasion, and the occurrence of metastasis. The revision includes grading (p. 14), staging (p. 32), and handling and reporting of the different types of specimens (p. 1).

Tissue Available for Study

Needle Core Biopsy

The grade and amount (number of positive cores and per cent of cancer). A minimum of three levels should be taken to enhance the detection of small foci of carcinoma. The sections should be spaced and mounted on three slides so that, in case a second opinion is desired or the patient is transferred to another centre for treatment, extra slides are available. If the urologist has indicated the site of each biopsy, relevant fragments should be separately mounted and labelled.

Transurethral Resection

Ideally, all pieces should be examined microscopically, but it has been recommended that a minimum of six cassettes for the first 10 g of tissue and one cassette for every 10 g of the remaining tissue be examined.[1]

Total Prostatectomy

The prostatectomy specimen should be examined externally. If fresh tissue is desired for special studies, e.g., DNA or RNA, biopsies should be taken and immediately frozen. The biopsy site should be inked before cutting and sutured after the biopsy has been taken to avoid false positive margins. The prostate should be suspended in fixative to maintain its shape. After fixation, the specimen should be weighed and measured and surfaces inked. The prostate should be sectioned at close intervals (3.5 mm) and the pieces should be numbered. Thicker sections may miss small tumours. If no tumour is grossly visible, random sections should be taken, particularly from the area reported to be positive in the biopsy. The unsampled specimen should be saved for later study.

Pathology Report on Total Prostatectomy

The pathology report on total prostatectomy specimens should include the following information: size and weight of the prostate, number of tumours, estimated volume and location, cell type, report of the highest grade, status of the surgical margin, presence of extra prostatic extension, presence of vascular and/or lymphatic invasion,

---

[1] Henson DE, Hutter RVP, Farrow GW (1994) Practice protocol for the examination of specimens removed from patients with carcinoma of the prostate gland. Arch Pathol Lab Med 118:779.

presence of neurovascular bundles and whether they are involved, and presence of prostatic intraepithelial neoplasia.

Categories of Prostate Carcinoma

Carcinoma of the prostate is commonly categorised as follows:
1. Clinical carcinoma: *A case in which a diagnosis of prostatic carcinoma is made clinically and confirmed by microscopic examination.*
2. Occult carcinoma: *Tumours that are manifested by their metastases before the primary site is detected.*
3. Other carcinomas: These are discovered incidentally, either at autopsy (latent carcinoma) or at surgery performed for unrelated disease (incidental carcinoma).

Histological Classification of Prostate Tumours

1   Epithelial Tumours

1.1   Benign
1.1.1   Papillary adenoma   8260/0[1]

1.2   Precursor lesion
1.2.1   Prostatic intraepithelial neoplasia   8148/2[2]

1.3   Malignant
1.3.1   Adenocarcinoma (carcinoma)   8140/3
1.3.1.1 Variants of adenocarcinoma
1.3.2   Urothelial (transitional cell) carcinoma   8120/3
1.3.3   Squamous cell carcinoma   8070/3
1.3.4   Basal cell carcinoma   8147/3
1.3.5   Small cell carcinoma   8041/3
1.3.6   Undifferentiated carcinoma   8020/3

2   Nonepithelial Tumours

2.1   Benign
2.2   Malignant
2.2.1   Rhabdomyosarcoma   8900/3
2.2.2   Leiomyosarcoma   8890/3
2.2.3   Stromal sarcoma   8935/3
2.2.4   Other Sarcomas

---

[1] Morphology code of the International Classification of Diseases for Oncology (ICD-O) and the Systematized Nomenclature of Medicine (SNOMED).
[2] 8148/2 applies only to prostatic intraepithelial neoplasia, grade III.

3   Miscellaneous Tumours

3.1   *Carcinoid tumour*   8240/3
3.2   *Carcinosarcoma*   8980/3
3.3   *Melanoma*   8720/3
3.4   *Phyllodes tumour*   9020/1
3.5   *Tumours of mesonephric tissue*   9110/1
3.6   *Paraganglioma*   8680/1

4   Secondary Tumours

5   Hematopoietic and Lymphoid Tumours

6   Unclassified Tumours

7   Epithelial Abnormalities

7.1   *Treatment effects*
7.1.1 *Cautery effect*
7.1.2 *Radiation therapy*
7.1.3 *Estrogen therapy*
7.1.4 *Antiandrogen therapy*
7.2   *Squamous metaplasia*
7.3   *Mucous metaplasia*
7.4   *Melanosis*

8   Tumour-like Lesions

8.1   *Atrophy*
8.2   *Hyperplasia*
8.2.1 *Atypical*
8.2.2 *Microacinar*
8.2.3 *Atypical glands*
8.2.4 *Cribriform*
8.2.5 *Basal cell*
8.2.6 *Sclerosing adenosis*
8.2.7 *Postatrophic*
8.2.8 *Reactive*
8.2.9 *Papillary*
8.2.10 *Stromal*
8.3   *Chronic prostatitis*

Definitions and Explanatory Notes

1 Epithelial Tumours

1.1 Benign

1.1.1 *Papillary adenoma* (Fig. 1)

A papillary tumour occurring in prostatic urethra composed of discrete fibrovascular papillary fronds lined by benign prostatic secretory cells.

Mitoses are rare. The lesion usually occurs in young men and cystoscopically presents as cherry red projections in the prostatic urethra. The distinction from the more common papillary hyperplasia is based on the presence of a more voluminous stromal core in the latter.

1.2 Precursor Lesion (Figs. 2–7)

1.2.1 *Prostatic intraepithelial neoplasia (PIN)*

Pre-existing acini and ducts lined by large cells with large nuclei containing one or more large nucleoli.

The neoplastic cells are confined to the acini or ducts. The nuclei show moderate to marked nuclear anaplasia. There is often intra-acinar and intraductal growth of cells, resulting in piling up of the epithelium, but the lining cells may be only one or two layers in thickness. The basal cell layer is demonstrable by basal cell-specific, monoclonal antibodies to high molecular weight keratin (e.g., 34βE12) or other markers (e.g., bcl-2, p63). It may be continuous or discontinuous. Occasionally, anaplasia may be manifested by nuclear features other than nucleoli, for example variation in nuclear size, shape, staining intensity, i.e., the features one generally associates with malignancy. PIN is not graded and the diagnosis is limited to the previously designated "high grade PIN". For lesions previously coded as "low grade prostatic intraepithelial neoplasia", see section 8.2.1.

1.3   Malignant

1.3.1   *Adenocarcinoma (carcinoma)* (Figs. 8–66)

An invasive malignant epithelial tumour consisting of secretory cells.
    The tumour shows various cell types, degrees of anaplasia and differentiation, immunohistochemical reactions, growth patterns, and invasive features. A diagnosis of malignancy may be based upon the presence of nuclear anaplasia, morphology of the glands, clear evidence that the glands are invasive, or any combination of these.

Nuclear anaplasia (Fig. 8)

Nuclear anaplasia is evidenced by the presence of nuclei that are often larger and more varied in shape than those of the adjacent, obviously benign glands. In most prostate carcinomas, the nuclei are fairly uniform. They may be vesicular, with coarse chromatin at the periphery. Their nucleoli may be larger than those of basal cells or benign hyperplastic glands. The nucleoli may be irregularly shaped and there may be more than one nucleolus. The presence of nucleoli is not essential for a diagnosis of prostate carcinoma, but they are usually present. Small nucleoli may be visible in benign secretory and basal cells, but this is without significance. Some carcinomas may show little or no anaplasia and the diagnosis is based on glandular morphology or invasive stromal dispersion.

Glandular morphology (Figs. 9–12)

Invasive glands often but not always have darker cytoplasm than adjacent benign glands. They usually show more variation in size and shape, with irregular or angulated contours and variable spacing between glands. Luminal mucin in irregular, dark-staining glands that are devoid of basal cells usually is indicative of carcinoma. However, neither crystalloids nor luminal mucin is diagnostic of malignancy when considered alone.

Invasive stromal dispersion (Figs. 13–22)

It is occasionally possible to recognise malignancy by the widespread dispersion of acini around and between benign glandular elements, although they will usually also exhibit some alteration of morphology and nuclear atypia. Vascular and lymphatic space invasion must be distinguished from retraction artefacts by the presence of an endothelial lining or by red blood cells or lymphocytes. Tumour in perineural spaces generally indicates invasive carcinoma, but it must be noted that benign glands may be in contact with nerves without denoting carcinoma. Circumferential involvement of the perineural space would represent perineural invasion. Glands without apparent nuclear anaplasia which appear to be in the perineural space should, to some degree, conform to the contour of the space before being interpreted as malignant when no other evidence of carcinoma is present. Extraprostatic invasion is evidenced by the presence of neoplastic glands in fibroadipose tissue devoid of smooth muscle fibres. Prostatic glands which are external to the prostate must be interpreted with caution, since normal glands are occasionally found in periprostatic fat. This is true also of skeletal muscle which is admixed with prostatic acini. Skeletal muscle is seen normally in the lateral and anterior regions of the prostate and it may contain benign glands. Invasion of the bladder neck is evidenced by the presence of neoplastic glands or individual carcinoma cells in vesical lamina propria or muscularis propria. Vascular invasion is not uncommon in this location.

If seminal vesicles are present, the presence of neoplastic glands should be sought and reported. Involutional changes in the seminal vesicles (p. 28) should not be misdiagnosed as carcinoma.

The minimum criterion for diagnosis of carcinoma is the finding of any of these three features: altered architecture, invasive growth pattern, or nuclear anaplasia. The presence of large nucleoli is the most important criterion for diagnosis of prostate carcinoma.

Cell types of prostate carcinoma (Figs. 23–28)

Heterogeneity of cell population is present in many prostate carcinomas. Several cell types are recognised by light microscopy – clear (i.e., pale or foamy), dark (slightly basophilic), and cells with distinctly granular and eosinophilic cytoplasm. The last are the paracrine-endocrine (neuroendocrine) cells, which are present normally in the glands, ducts, and prostatic urethra. They may be recognised by their eosinophilic granules, but immunohistochemistry is usually needed. They produce one or more paracrine-endocrine substances and sometimes prostatic acid phosphatase (PAP) and prostate-specific antigen (PSA). Approximately 10% of prostatic adenocarcinoma have extensive or multifocal areas with neuroendocrine differentiation but, except for the small cell carcinomas (see 1.3.5 below), the clinical significance of this is uncertain. It is recommended that the presence of neuroendocrine differentiation and an estimate of its extent be noted in pathology reports for the purpose of future study.

Some cells may have an oncocytic or vacuolated appearance.

Immunohistochemical (IHC) analysis (Figs. 29–35)

In normal and hyperplastic glands, the secretory cells lining the acini, prostatic ducts, and prostatic urethra show a uniformly strong positive reaction for both PAP and PSA. Prostate carcinomas react positively with antibodies to both PAP and PSA, but the intensity varies. Transitional epithelium of the prostatic ducts and urethra, the basal cells of prostatic acini, the epithelium of the ejaculatory ducts, and the seminal vesicles do not react with PAP and PSA. PAP is positive in carcinoids, particularly of the rectum.

Basal cell-specific high molecular weight keratin (e.g., 34βE12) is helpful to identify lesions confined to ducts or acini and to distinguish between invasive carcinoma and prostatic intraepithelial neoplasia. It should be noted that some benign glands lack basal cells and keratins are not informative if the pathologist has not first determined that the cells are malignant. The neuroendocrine cells may be studied immunochemically for the presence of various peptides (chromogranin, synaptophysin, serotonin, calcitonin, etc.). Immunohistochemistry may be helpful in identifying residual neoplastic cells following therapy (see p. 32).

Other markers such as prostatic-specific membrane antigen (PSMA) have been and are being developed at present, but PAP and PSA are the most commonly utilised markers.

In well-differentiated prostate carcinoma, a positive reaction for PAP and PSA is demonstrable in most cells. Papillary tumours show a strong positive reaction often in the apical cytoplasm of secretory cells. Poorly differentiated and undifferentiated prostate carcinomas in which hematoxylin and eosin stains show homogeneous staining are often quite heterogeneous with PAP and PSA. Although some tumours are strongly positive in most cells, others show only individual cells or clones that are positive. A rare tumour is negative for one or the other and sometimes for both. Often it is the PSA that is negative.

Variants of growth patterns (Figs. 36–42)

Most prostate carcinomas form glands which manifest one or more of the following patterns. Frequently more than one growth pattern is seen in an individual case.

Acinar (Figs. 36, 37)

An invasive carcinoma composed of secretory cells showing a variable degree of nuclear anaplasia devoid of basal cells and forming acini.

The latter are of variable size but are usually smaller than benign glands. They are simple in structure and without convolutions. Rarely, the acini are very small. Tumours consisting entirely of simple small or large glands are categorised as well-differentiated.

Cribriform (Fig. 38)

A large acinar tumour in which the neoplastic cells show bridging across the lumen without intervening stroma.

This is categorised as a moderately differentiated tumour.

Fused gland (Fig. 39)

Groups of acini are packed closely together without intervening stroma.

Tumours showing fused gland patterns are categorised as poorly differentiated tumours. These differ from cribriform glands in that they are more cellular and their peripheral contours are irregular. At low power, the volume of the cells exceeds that of the luminal spaces.

Solid/trabecular (Figs. 40, 41)

Cells are arranged in sheets, trabeculae, or cords devoid of acinar differentiation.

These tumours are also categorised as poorly differentiated.

Papillary (Fig. 42)

Neoplastic cells, usually stratified, line papillary fronds.

The cells may be cuboidal and the cytoplasm is granular. Because these were originally believed to arise in the utricle (which is of Müllerian origin), they were designated as endometrioid or ductal carcinomas. However, they are now known to occur elsewhere in the prostate, particularly in the prostatic urethra, the adjacent ducts, or deeper within the prostate and in cystic areas. There is often typical carcinoma elsewhere in the prostate.

Grading of Prostate Carcinoma

Many grading systems have been proposed for prostate adenocarcinoma. Two systems will be described.

Gleason grading (Figs. 43–50)

The Gleason grading system[1] is based on growth patterns. The most prevalent pattern is designated as the primary pattern and the second most prevalent is designated as secondary. Each pattern is given one of five numbers. The primary pattern is added to the secondary one to give the Gleason score. If only one pattern is seen, the score is derived by doubling the number.

The Gleason grading system:

Pattern 1.   Single, separate, uniform glands closely packed, with definite edge

Pattern 2.   Single, separate uniform glands loosely packed, with irregular edge

Pattern 3A. Single, separate, uniform glands, scattered

Pattern 3B. Single, separate, very small glands, scattered

Pattern 3C. Papillary/cribriform masses, smoothly circumscribed

Pattern 4A. Fused glands, raggedly infiltrating

Pattern 4B. Same, with large pale cells ("hypernephroid")

Pattern 5A. Almost solid, rounded masses, necrosis ("comedocarcinoma")

Pattern 5B. Anaplastic, raggedly infiltrating.

This system is undergoing modifications.

---

[1] Gleason DF (1977) Histologic grading and clinical staging of prostatic carcinoma. In: Tannenbaum M (ed) Urologic pathology: the prostate. Lea and Febiger, Philadelphia, pp 171–97.

World Health Organization Grading System (Figs. 51–56)

This system is based on the degrees of nuclear anaplasia and glandular differentiation.

Degrees of nuclear anaplasia (Figs. 51–53)

Mild anaplasia (Fig. 51)

The nuclei are fairly uniform with minimal variation in size and shape. They are very similar to those of benign glands with minimal discernible anaplastic features. A few nucleoli may be present, but the diagnosis of carcinoma is based chiefly on morphology or invasive dispersion of the acini.

Moderate anaplasia (Fig. 52)

The characteristic feature of moderate nuclear anaplasia is the presence of many prominent nucleoli, readily seen on medium power.

Marked anaplasia (Fig. 53)

The nuclei show marked variation in size and shape. They may be hyperchromatic but more often they are vesicular and irregularly shaped and are two to three times larger than adjacent benign nuclei. Mitotic figures are, generally speaking, rare in carcinoma of the prostate, but with marked anaplasia they may be numerous and even abnormal.

In arriving at a WHO grade, the three degrees of anaplasia are counted as I, II, or III.

Degrees of glandular differentiation (Figs. 54–56)

Since normal prostate consists of glands, the WHO grading system regards the tumours that form glands as well-differentiated and those with few or no glands as poorly differentiated. Histological scoring assigns a numerical score of 1–5 depending on the type and amount of glandular differentiation.

Well-differentiated tumours consist of simple small or large glands. Moderately differentiated ones consist of cribriform glands. Poorly differentiated tumours show little or no gland formation. In arriving at the WHO grade, degrees of differentiation are counted as follows:

1. All of the tumour is composed of well-differentiated elements.
2. The tumour is composed of at least some moderately differentiated elements. Well-differentiated elements may or may not be present.
3. The tumour has poorly differentiated elements, but these are estimated to comprise less than 15% of the tumour.
4. The tumour has poorly differentiated elements that are estimated to comprise between 16% and 25% of the tumour.
5. The tumour has poorly differentiated elements that are estimated to comprise over 25% of the tumour.

The WHO grade of the tumour is the sum of the anaplasia and differentiation values. For example: If the nuclear grade is II and histologic grade is 3, the WHO grade is 5. If nuclear grade is III and histologic grade is 5, the WHO grade is 8.

1.3.1.1 Variants of adenocarcinoma (Figs. 57–66)

A variety of cell types occur and should be incorporated into the diagnosis for future study and comparison of different treatment modalities. Some invasive carcinomas simulate the morphology of hyperplastic or atrophic glands and are distinguished by their invasive dispersion or nuclear anaplasia. Some are associated with dense lymphocytic infiltrate. Hyaline globules likely represent remote mucin deposits (Figs. 57–61.

Mucinous carcinoma (Figs. 62–63)

A carcinoma with ample amounts of extracellular mucin.

Some luminal mucin is present in many prostate carcinomas, but this designation is reserved for tumours that are principally mucinous and show stromal extravasation. A secondary carcinoma such as one extending from the colon must be ruled out. The true nature of the tumour can be identified readily by PAP and PSA, both of which are positive.

Spindle cell carcinoma (Fig. 64)

A rare carcinoma that contains spindle cells resembling a sarcoma.

The change may be encountered in treated carcinomas and usually is associated with focal areas of differentiated carcinoma.

Prostate carcinoma with ectopic placental glycoprotein production (Figs. 65, 66)
A high-grade carcinoma with bizarre mononuclear or multinuclear cells sometimes resembling syncytiotrophoblasts that react positively with placental glycoproteins. Unlike choriocarcinoma, immunoreactivity is seen in both the large cells and small cells.

1.3.2   Urothelial (transitional cell) carcinoma (Fig. 67)

A prostate tumour composed of urothelial cells.
These carcinomas of the bladder or urethra may invade into the prostate stroma directly. They may also originate in the prostate ducts or extend into them from the urethra. The prostate stroma may subsequently be infiltrated from tumour in the ducts. Occasionally, there is a coincidental prostatic adenocarcinoma.

1.3.3   Squamous cell carcinoma (Fig. 68)

An uncommon tumour with squamous cell differentiation.
Squamous elements may be seen in prostatic adenocarcinoma, usually due to treatment. These should be classified as prostatic adenocarcinoma with squamous differentiation.

1.3.4   Basal cell carcinoma (Figs. 69, 70)

A malignant tumour of prostatic basal cells.
The growth generally has a similarity to typical basal cell hyperplasia but is more diffuse and includes cellular anaplasia, sheets of poorly differentiated cells, mitoses, tumour necrosis or other characteristics of malignancy. There may be focal areas of squamous, transitional, and acinar differentiation. If these features are equivocal, a malignant diagnosis may be based upon the presence of extraprostatic invasion. These tumours are rare.

1.3.5   *Small cell carcinoma* (Figs. 71, 72)

A malignant tumour identical to small cell carcinoma of the lung.

Prostatic carcinoma may also be demonstrated, and lacking this element, metastatic disease must be considered, as well as extension from a primary bladder small cell carcinoma.

Synonyms: small cell neuroendocrine carcinoma, oat cell carcinoma

1.3.6   *Undifferentiated carcinoma* (Fig. 73)

A malignant tumour that is too poorly differentiated to be placed in any other category.

2   Nonepithelial Tumours

These are named and defined according to the WHO Histological Classification of Soft Tissue Tumours.[1]

2.1   Benign

It is questionable whether true leiomyomas and fibromas of the prostate exist. The commonly encountered, circumscribed masses of smooth muscle and/or fibrous tissue are considered to be hyperplastic rather than neoplastic.

2.2   Malignant

Prostatic sarcomas are uncommon. A variety of types occur. Only those with any appreciable frequency are listed.

---

[1] Weiss SW (1994) World Health Organization histological typing of soft tissue tumours, second edn. Springer, Heidelberg.

2.2.1   *Rhabdomyosarcoma* (Fig. 74)

A malignant tumour of skeletal muscle that resembles those seen elsewhere

2.2.2   *Leiomyosarcoma* (Fig. 75)

A tumour of smooth muscle cells resembling tumours seen in other locations.

2.2.3   *Stromal sarcoma* (Figs. 76, 77)

A rare malignant mesenchymal tumour composed of undifferentiated spindle cells that do not show myogenous differentiation.

2.2.4   *Others*

3   Miscellaneous Tumours

3.1   Carcinoid tumour

3.2   *Carcinosarcoma* (Fig. 78)

A rare tumour containing both malignant epithelial and malignant heterologous mesenchymal elements. The sarcomatous component must be identifiable as a specific sarcoma, e.g., rhabdomyo-, osteo-, or chondrosarcoma.

Synonym: malignant mixed mesodermal tumour

3.3   Melanoma (Fig. 79)

A rare tumour that is histologically, biologically, and immunohistochemically identical to melanomas seen elsewhere.

When primary melanoma of prostate is suspected, certain criteria should be met: negative history of prior melanoma of the skin, eye, or other sites. Examination of all skin surfaces should be negative. The distribution of any metastatic deposits should be consistent with that of a primary prostate neoplasm.

3.4   Phyllodes Tumour (Figs. 80–82)

A prostatic tumour consisting of a stromal proliferation with bizarre nuclei and a glandular component that is often cystic, linear, or associated with polyps.

Occasionally the stromal elements may be very cellular. By contrast, stromal hyperplasia and stromal sarcomas do not show an abnormal glandular element. The lesion tends to recur. As in the breast, it may be difficult to predict the ultimate outcome, so the term phyllodes is more appropriate than cystosarcoma phyllodes. Occasionally the stromal element is clearly malignant.

3.5   Tumours of Mesonephric Tissue (Fig. 83)

Primary benign or malignant tumours of the prostate that consist of mesonephric tissues: when malignant, this resembles Wilms tumour.

3.6   Paraganglioma

Paraganglioma of the prostate is identical to those occurring elsewhere.

Synonym: phaeochromocytoma

4   Secondary Tumours (Fig. 84)

Metastatic tumours and tumours extending into the prostate from adjacent organs such as the bladder, the prostatic urethra, and the rectum.

5   Hematopoietic and Lymphoid Tumours (Fig. 85)

This category applies to tumours initially manifested as prostate tumour. Lymphomas of the prostate do not differ from those seen elsewhere. The neoplastic cells are generally of B cell type, but any type may occur. These and the leukemias, however, must be distinguished from the far more common infiltrates of chronic prostatitis. The former shows a random pattern of spread through the prostatic stroma with dissection of the fibromuscular tissue and only occasional con-

tact with glandular elements. The epithelium of the glands is not usually altered. In prostatitis, the mononuclear infiltrate uniformly exhib-
its an affinity for glandular and ductal elements and produces an alteration of glandular epithelium: it becomes ulcerated, atrophic, squamous, or proliferative and the tall columnar secretory epithelium is
attenuated or absent.

6   Unclassified Tumours

*Benign or malignant tumours that can not be placed in any of the cat-
egories described above.*

7   Epithelial Alterations

7.1   Treatment Effects

Cautery and treatment by radiation, estrogens, antiandrogens, or other medications may alter the appearance of normal or neoplastic epithelium.

7.1.1   *Cautery effect* (Fig. 86)

The cautery effect on prostate cells, whether benign or malignant, re-
sults in elongated cells with hyperchromatic nuclei simulating transitional cell carcinoma. Additional sections and immunohistochemistry
often reveal the true nature of the findings.

7.1.2   *Radiation therapy* (Figs. 87–89)

The cytoplasm of the tumour cells is vacuolated and increased in volume and the cell membranes are lost. The nuclei are enlarged, chromatin is clumped, and nuclei may be pyknotic or sometimes bizarre.
The tumour-free prostate shows atrophy of secretory epithelium, nuclear atypia, and occasionally some squamoid metaplasia.

7.1.3   *Estrogen therapy* (Figs. 90, 91)

The cytoplasm of the glandular epithelium is clear and there is rupture of cell membranes. The nuclei are reduced in size by approximately 50%. There are pyknosis and loss of nucleoli. In the non-neoplastic glands, there is atrophy of glandular epithelium and squamous metaplasia of the ducts.

7.1.4   *Antiandrogen therapy* (Figs. 92–95)

Residual tumour cells may exist only as smudged, cell-shaped pale deposits within the stroma. Some tumour glands show loss of cell membranes, reduction of cell size following dissolution of cytoplasm, and resultant crowding together of the residual acinar nuclei. Cell loss may produce cystic spaces.

Immunohistochemistry may be useful for identifying residual tumour cells, e.g., wide-spectrum cytokeratin, PSMA, and maspin. PAP/PSA may not be present. Tumours that exhibit such cellular changes should not be graded. A statement should be made as to the degree and extent of treatment effect. Benign elements of the prostate become atrophic, the basal cells become unusually prominent, and the glands sometimes contain squamous cell aggregates

7.2   Squamous Metaplasia (Fig. 96)

Benign squamous cells replacing the ductal and/or acinar epithelial cells.

Squamous metaplasia occurs as solid nests. The cells are well differentiated and show neither anaplasia, mitoses, nor evidence of invasion. Squamous metaplasia is associated with infarction and may be seen in acini and/or ducts of older men, possibly representing healed infarcts or ischemia.

7.3   Mucous Metaplasia (Fig. 97)

Benign glands lined by mucous-producing epithelial cells.

The lesion has a striking resemblance to the cells of Cowper glands except that the glandular morphology is typically prostatic.

7.4   Melanosis (Fig. 98)

A deposition of melanin pigment in prostatic secretory cells with or without similar deposits in prostatic stroma.

This rare lesion is without known significance. It may involve benign or malignant prostatic cells. Melanin confined to stromal cells constitutes the blue naevus (see 8.6 below).

8   Tumour-Like Lesions

8.1   Atrophy (Figs. 99–101)

The glands are small and have a lobular arrangement around a central duct. They are lined by small cells with scant cytoplasm. The cells react positively with high molecular weight keratin. The nuclei are small and dark-staining. They appear close together like a string of pearls. The adjacent stroma may show sclerosis. In contrast, in small acinar prostate carcinoma the epithelial cells usually have considerable cytoplasm, the nuclei are larger and more vesicular, and there may be prominent nucleoli. Atrophic glands may be cystic.

8.2   Hyperplasia (Fig. 102)

In contrast to the uniformity seen in normal glands, hyperplastic glands show considerable variation in structural appearance. Varying degrees of glandular and stromal hyperplasia are seen. Usually the acini are enlarged and papillary processes of epithelium project into the lumina. Two cell types are seen, the secretory and the basal cells. The former may be columnar or cuboidal. The cells have poorly defined borders. The cytoplasm is finely granular or homogeneous. The nuclei are round and vesicular and may have small nucleoli. There is often a basal layer of cells which are low cuboidal with small vesicular nuclei and which may contain small nucleoli. The acini are round or elongated and have a regular outline surrounded by loose fibromuscular stroma.

8.2.1   Atypical hyperplasia (Fig. 103)

Pre-existing glands display some atypical nuclear changes in the secretory cells which fall short of changes sufficient for a diagnosis of prostatic intraepithelial neoplasia.

This is the lesion previously designated as "low grade intraepithelial neoplasia".

8.2.2   Microacinar hyperplasia (Figs. 104, 105)

Simple, small glands often located at the periphery of hyperplastic nodules or possibly comprising the whole nodule.

The presence of small closely packed acini lined by a single layer of cells suggests prostate carcinoma, but no nuclear anaplasia or dispersion of glands is seen.

Synonyms: atypical adenomatous hyperplasia (AAH), adenosis.

8.2.3   Atypical glands (Fig. 106–108)

This term refers to aggregates of small glands lined by a single layer of cells (i.e., an absence of the basal cell layer). In such cases, the differential diagnosis is of small acinar prostate carcinoma or microacinar hyperplasia. When there is any doubt as to whether invasive dispersion and/or nuclear anaplasia is present, the lesion is classified as atypical glands, whether they occur as single glands or aggregates of glands.

Synonym: atypical small acinar proliferation

8.2.4   Cribriform hyperplasia (Figs. 109, 110)

Gland-in-gland growth or bridging of the cells. Nuclei are uniform and nucleoli are very small, usually absent.

There will usually be a layer of basal cells but, unlike PIN with a cribriform pattern of proliferation, the secretory cells are completely normal. In cribriform carcinoma, peripheral contours are variably irregular, the basal cells are absent, and the nuclei are often pyknotic toward the centre. The nucleoli are usually prominent in the periphery and there is likely to be obvious glandular carcinoma elsewhere.

8.2.5   Basal cell hyperplasia (Figs. 111–114)

Tubular or acinar structures containing cells that are small and of uniform size with scant cytoplasm. Small nucleoli and occasional mitoses may be present.

The cell nests have a distinct outline. Basal cell hyperplasia may involve single or multiple acini occurring in aggregates, focally or diffusely distributed. The cell nests may form acini with lumina or appear as solid nests. In most basal cell hyperplasias, there is usually some secretory differentiation of luminal cells, which is best demonstrated by the prostatic acid phosphatase or prostatic specific antigen. Occasionally, squamous change may be seen. In some cases, basal cells form anastomosing cords one to two cell layers thick. In others, they form masses surrounding circular spaces. This group has a lobular pattern and may be misinterpreted as adenoid cystic carcinoma. In basal cell hyperplasia, the cells usually give a positive reaction to 34βE12. The adjacent stroma often shows increased cellularity.

Synonym: foetalisation of the prostate, basal cell adenoma

8.2.6   Sclerosing adenosis (Figs. 115–118)

Nodules of hyperplastic stroma with small, irregularly distributed glands that often are surrounded by a thick basement membrane.

This is the only type of hyperplasia that shows true myoepithelial cells, giving a positive reaction for actin, S-100 protein, and keratin.

Synonym: fibroglandular nodule

8.2.7   Postatrophic hyperplasia (Fig. 119)

Lobular distribution of atrophic glands side by side with glands that have considerably more cytoplasm and normal-appearing nuclei.

Synonym: partial atrophy

8.2.8   Reactive hyperplasia (Fig. 120)

The glands have a cribriform or bridging growth pattern admixed with inflammatory cells. This is a reactive process encountered in chronic prostatitis.

The periacinar inflammatory infiltrate should lead to the correct diagnosis.

8.2.9   *Papillary hyperplasia* (Fig. 121)

A benign proliferation of prostatic secretory epithelium which projects into the prostatic urethra or into cystic spaces
Unlike papillary adenomas (p. 9) in which the fronds have delicate fibrovascular cores, these lesions have more abundant stroma with variably papillary/polypoid contours. The nuclei are bland.

8.2.10   *Stromal hyperplasia* (Fig. 122)

Nodular or diffuse proliferation of prostate stroma.
This proliferation may be fibrous, myomatous, or both.

8.3   Chronic Prostatitis (Figs. 123, 124)

Occasionally, the infiltrating lymphocytes of chronic prostatitis have vacuolisation mimicking signet ring cells or peripheral halos mimicking clear cell carcinoma. The cells do not form glandular structures and are PAP- and PSA-negative. See p. 20 for comparison of prostatitis and lymphoma.

8.4   Granulomatous Prostatitis

8.4.1   *Nonspecific granulomatous prostatitis* (Figs. 125–127)

A localised, lobular, granulomatous inflammation with lymphocytes, plasma cells, multinucleated giant cells, and epithelioid histiocytes lacking a specific aetiology.
The lesion is associated with a destroyed duct or acinus. In the earliest stages, the lesion consists of dilated ducts and acini containing neutrophils, foamy histiocytes, and debris. This differs from specific granulomatous prostatitis in that no specific causal agent is demonstrable and the granuloma is centred around destroyed acini and is non-necrotic. Digital rectal examination may suggest a carcinoma because the prostate is hard. Nonspecific necrotising granulomas are seen at the site of prior transurethral resections.

8.4.2   *Specific granulomatous prostatitis* (Figs. 128–131)

Granulomatous prostatitis in which a specific aetiologic agent can be demonstrated. Most common are those associated with acid-fast organisms following Calmette-Guérin bacillus therapy for superficial bladder carcinoma.

The lesion is similar to that seen elsewhere. Less common lesions are those of latent *Cryptococcus* and other fungi. Granulomas similar to those seen in systemic disease such as Churg-Straus syndrome (allergic granulomas) or Wegener's granulomatosis may rarely be seen in the prostate.

8.4.3   *Malakoplakia* (Figs. 132, 133)

Aggregates of eosinophilic macrophages with characteristic cytoplasmic inclusions.

Lymphocytes and plasma cells are usually present, but most of the cells are large, eosinophilic macrophages. A variable number of these von Hansemann histiocytes contain Michaelis-Gutmann inclusions. These are spherical, 5–8-μ bodies with a targetoid or bull's eye appearance that may be highlighted with stains for iron, calcium, or the periodic acid-Schiff reaction. This shows a periglandular location similar to nonspecific granulomatous prostatitis.

8.5   Myofibroblastic Proliferation

8.5.1   *Postoperative spindle cell nodule* (Fig. 134)

A proliferation of myofibroblasts at the site of a prior surgical procedure.

An exuberant, friable mass of tissue which develops usually within 1 to 3 months after the surgery. The centre of the lesion may contain only amorphous fibrinoid material and/or necrotic epithelial and stromal elements. Similar lesions are seen following needle biopsy as an irregular stellate defect surrounded by fibrosis. Periprostatic tissue may show fibrosis and hemosiderin deposition. Immunohistochemical reactivity of myofibroblasts distinguish these from spindled carcinomas. Frequent cytokeratin reactivity and the tissue culture growth pattern are helpful in distinguishing these from leiomyosarcoma.

Synonym: inflammatory pseudotumour.

8.6   Naevus (Fig. 135)

Infiltration of the fibrovascular stroma by stellate and spindle-shaped cells containing finely granular brown pigment in the cytoplasm.

The cells are distributed diffusely either in clumps or as single cells with elongated, branching cytoplasmic processes. The brown pigment may obscure the nuclei. Histochemically and immunochemically, these react as naevi elsewhere.

Synonym: blue naevus, stromal melanosis

8.7   Nephrogenic Adenoma (Fig. 136)

A non-neoplastic epithelial lesion consisting of cuboidal cells and tubules in the prostate.

The tubules are small and lined by small uniform cuboidal cells. There may also be microcysts lined by hobnail cells and mucin-producing cells resembling signet ring cells. These and the tubular lesions often have prominent basement membranes that distinguish this from carcinoma. The adjacent stroma is often inflammatory with lymphocytes and plasma cells. The lesion is seen usually near the urethra and may be misinterpreted as prostate carcinoma. They are negative for PAP/PSA.

8.8   Cowper Gland (Fig. 137)

Small round acini lined by low columnar mucin-containing epithelium and surrounding a central duct. The nuclei are small, basal, and uniform

8.9   Involutional Changes of Seminal Vesicle (Fig. 138)

Epithelium of seminal vesicle often has cells with large hyperchromatic nuclei that can be mistaken for malignancy. Many cells have golden brown lipofuscin pigment.

8.10   Endometriosis (Fig. 139)

Endometriosis in the prostate is identical to endometriosis seen elsewhere. This may occur after hormonal therapy.

8.11   Utricular Cysts (Fig. 140)

8.11.1   Utricular cysts

Utricular cysts are located in the verumontanum. The wall may be lined by columnar, cuboidal, transitional, or squamous cells or it may lack an epithelial lining.

8.11.2   Müllerian cysts

Müllerian cysts are located outside the prostate, between the prostate and the bladder. They are midline cysts. Occasionally these may be associated with other congenital anomalies, e.g., renal agenesis or dysgenesis, and abnormalities of external genitalia.

8.11.3   Retention cysts

Retention cysts are lined by flattened prostatic epithelium or transitional epithelium. The cysts are usually unilateral and found adjacent to the urethra.

8.11.4   Megacystic prostate (Fig. 141)

Enlarged prostate secondary to grossly evident cysts. The luminal epithelium is the prostatic secretory type and may or may not be malignant.

8.11.5   Post-therapy cyst (Fig. 142)

Following hormonal or antiandrogen therapy, there may be massive loss of neoplastic cells, leaving cystic spaces. There are usually residual neoplastic cells at the periphery of the space.

Tumours and Tumour-Like Lesions of Seminal Vesicles

1   Epithelial tumours

1.1   Adenofibroma (Figs. 143, 144)   8140/0

Ductal structures forming a benign neoplasm supported by stromal elements.
     It can be difficult to distinguish this from hyperplasia.

1.2   Adenocarcinoma (Fig. 145)   8140/3

A rare epithelial neoplasm usually forming ductal structures that can be demonstrated both grossly and microscopically to be of seminal vesicle origin.
     Many tumours diagnosed as carcinoma of the seminal vesicles are in fact carcinomas of the prostate. True carcinomas of the seminal vesicle have a tubulopapillary morphology, sometimes with brown pigment. PAP and PSA are negative. The tumour should form a dominant mass within the seminal vesicle.

2   Nonepithelial tumours

These are defined according to the WHO Histological Classification of Soft Tissue Tumours.[1] Fibromas and leiomyomas are the most frequently encountered tumours.

3   Tumour-like lesions

3.1   Involutional changes (Fig. 138) (see section 8.9, p. 28)

3.2   Amyloidosis (Fig. 146)

A diffuse deposition of amyloid replacing the stroma adjacent to seminal vesicle epithelium. This is without known clinical significance and is not associated with amyloidosis elsewhere.

---

[1] Weiss SW (1994) World Health Organization histological typing of soft tissue tumours, second edn. Springer, Heidelberg.

3.3 ' Cysts

Congenital cysts are usually unilateral, unilocular, and associated with ipsilateral renal agenesis or dysgenesis, occasionally with absence of the testis or cysts of the rete testis. The cyst may assume a large size. It contains white viscous fluid resembling secretions of seminal vesicle.

Acquired cysts are secondary to obstruction or inflammation of the seminal vesicles or ejaculatory ducts.

TNM Classification of Tumours of Prostate Carcinoma*

Rules for Classification

The classification applies only to adenocarcinomas. Transitional cell carcinoma of the prostate is classified as a urothelial tumour. There should be histological confirmation of the disease.

The following are the procedures for assessing T, N, and M categories:

T categories	Physical examination, imaging, endoscopy, biopsy, and biochemical tests.
N categories	Physical examination and imaging.
M categories	Physical examination, imaging, skeletal studies, and biochemical tests.

Regional Lymph Nodes

The regional lymph nodes are the nodes of the true pelvis, which essentially are the pelvic nodes below the bifurcation of the common iliac arteries. Laterality does not affect the N classification.

TNM Clinical Classification

T – Primary Tumour

TX	Primary tumour cannot be assessed
T0	No evidence of primary tumour
T1	Clinically inapparent tumour not palpable or visible by imaging

---

* Sobin LH, Wittekind CH (eds) (1997) TNM classification of malignant tumours, fifth edn. Wiley, New York.

T1a	Tumour incidental histological finding in 5% or less tissue resected
T1b	Tumour incidental histological finding in more than 5% of tissue resected
T1c	Tumour identified by needle biopsy[1] (e.g., because of elevated serum level of PSA)
T2	Tumour confined within the prostate[1]
T2a	Tumour involves one lobe
T2b	Tumour involves both lobes
T3	Tumour extends through the prostatic capsule
T3a	Extracapsular extension (unilateral or bilateral)
T3b	Tumour invades seminal vesicle(s)
T4	Tumour is fixed or invades adjacent structures other than seminal vesicles: bladder neck, external sphincter, rectum, levator muscles, and/or pelvic wall

N – Regional Lymph Nodes

NX	Regional lymph nodes cannot be assessed
N0	No regional lymph node metastasis
N1	Regional lymph node metastasis

M – Distant Metastasis

MX	Distant metastasis cannot be assessed
M0	No distant metastasis
M1	Distant metastasis
M1a	Nonregional lymph node(s)
M1b	Bone(s)
M1c	Other site(s)

Note: When metastasis is present in more than one site, the most advanced category should be used.

TNM Pathological Classification

The pT, pN, and pM categories correspond to T, N, and M categories. However, there is no pT1 category because there is insufficient tissue to assess the highest pT category.

---

[1] Tumour found in one or both lobes by needle biopsy but not palpable or visible by imaging is classified as T1c. Invasion into the prostatic apex or into (but not beyond) the prostatic capsule is not classified as T3 but as T2.

G – Histopathological Grading

GX   Grade cannot be assessed
G1   Well-differentiated (slight anaplasia)
G2   Moderately differentiated (moderate anaplasia)
G3–4   Poorly differentiated/undifferentiated (marked anaplasia)

Stage Grouping

Stage I

T1a	N0	M0	G1

Stage II

T1a	N0	M0	G2, 3–4
T1b	N0	M0	Any G
T1c	N0	M0	Any G
T1	N0	M0	Any G
T2	N0	M0	Any G

Stage III

T3	N0	M0	Any G

Stage IV

T4	N0	M0	Any G
Any T	N1	M0	Any G
Any T	Any N	M1	Any G

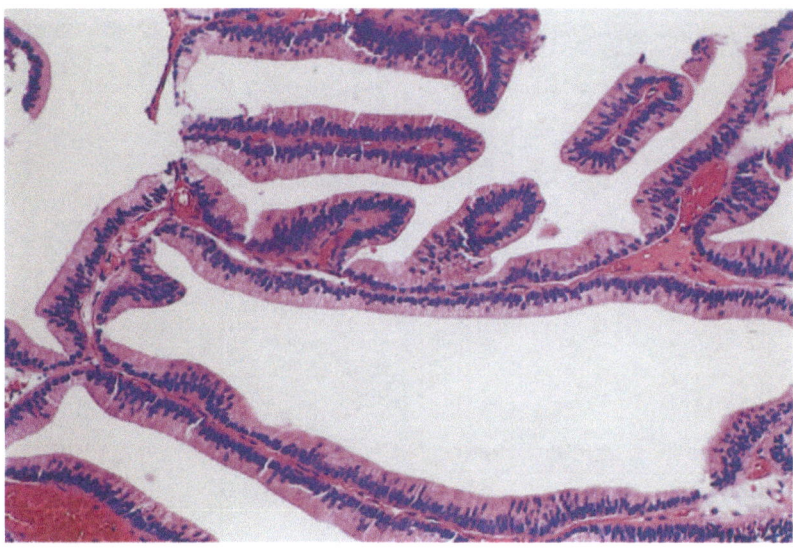

Fig. 1. Papillary adenoma

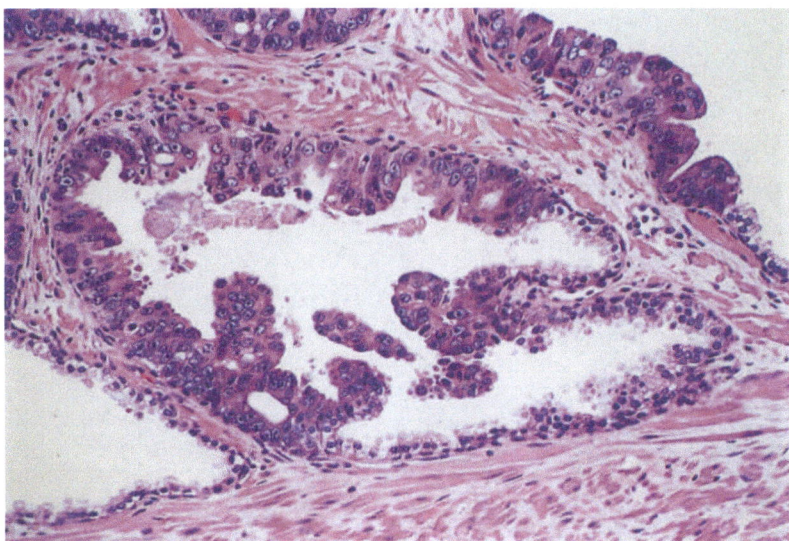

Fig. 2. Prostatic intraepithelial neoplasia

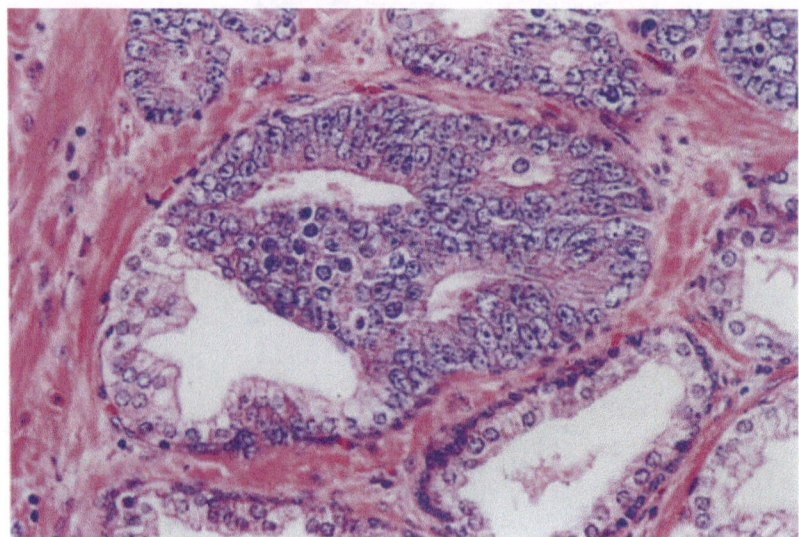

Fig. 3. Prostatic intraepithelial neoplasia with bridging

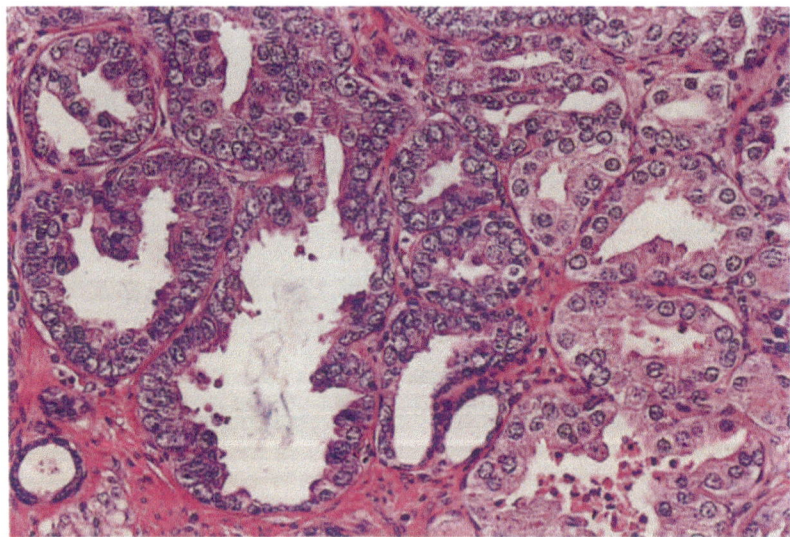

Fig. 4. Prostatic intraepithelial neoplasia resembling carcinoma

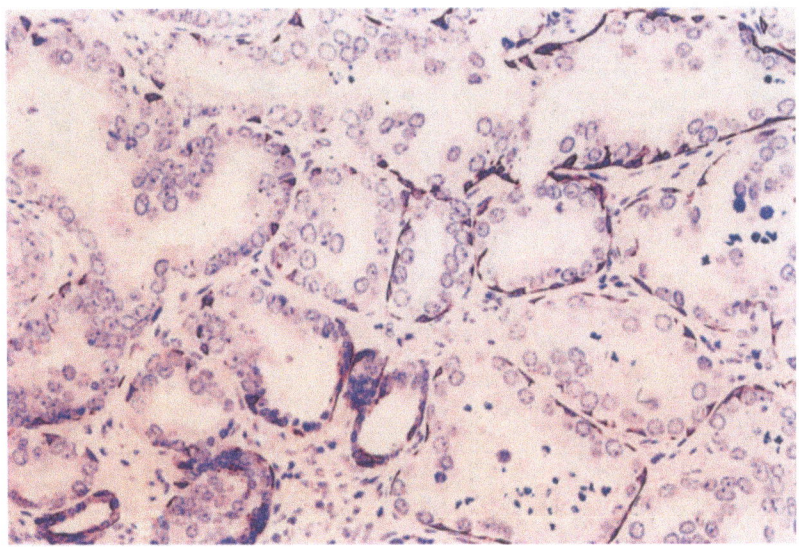

Fig. 5. Prostatic intraepithelial neoplasia with high molecular weight anti-keratin (34βE12). Same field as Fig. 4

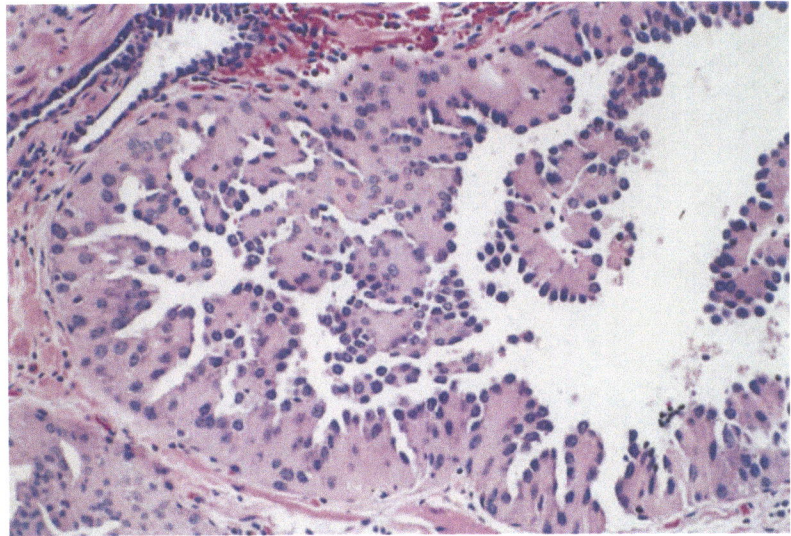

Fig. 6. Prostatic intraepithelial neoplasia, papillary pattern

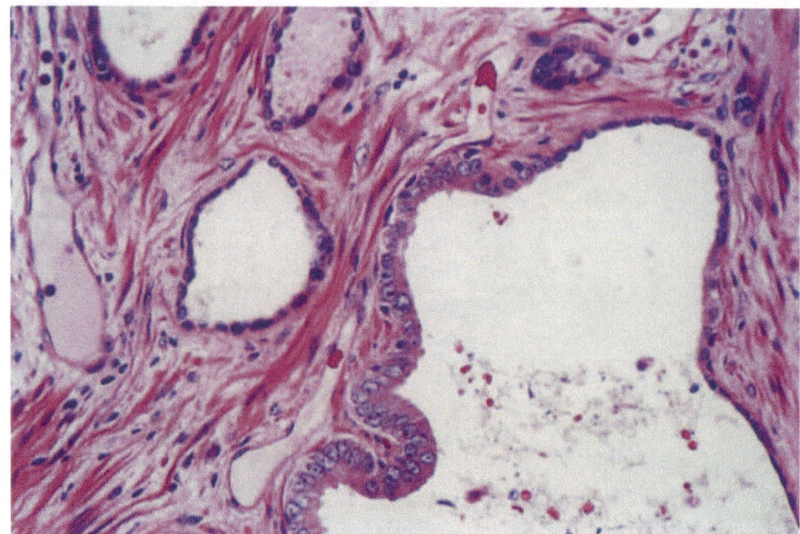

Fig. 7. Prostatic intraepithelial neoplasia involving atrophic glands

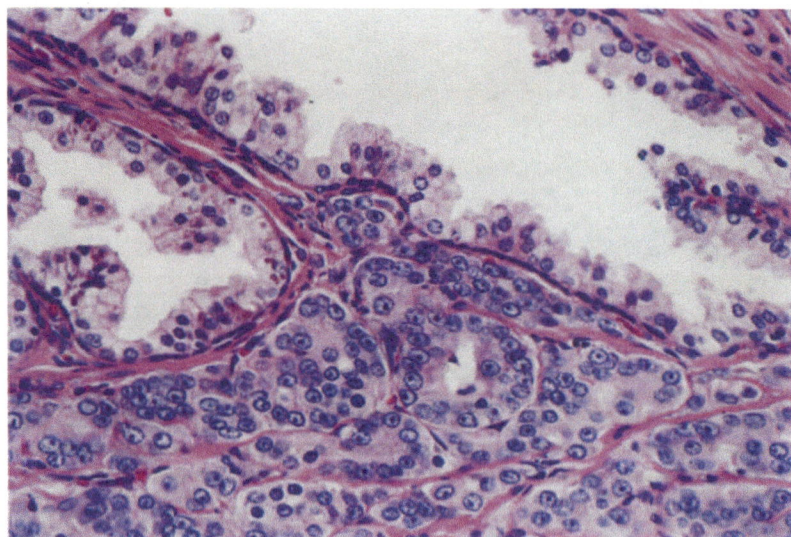

Fig. 8. Adenocarcinoma with nuclear anaplasia

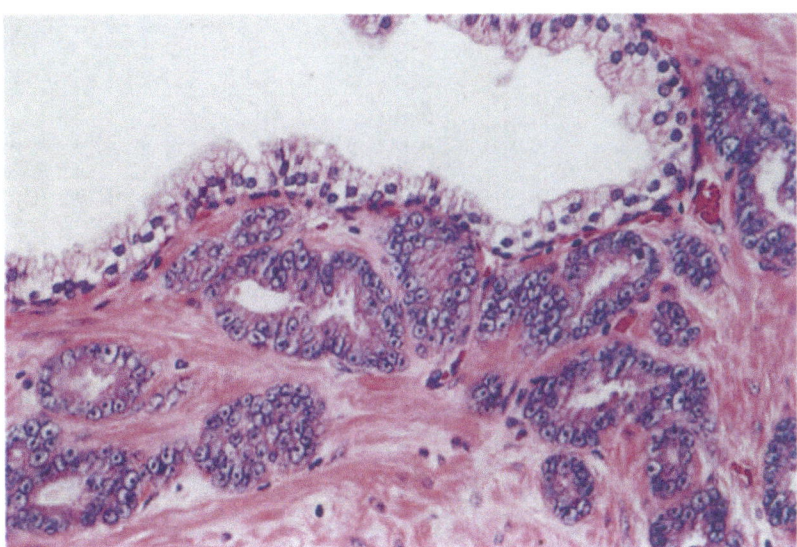

Fig. 9. Adenocarcinoma with amphophilic cytoplasm

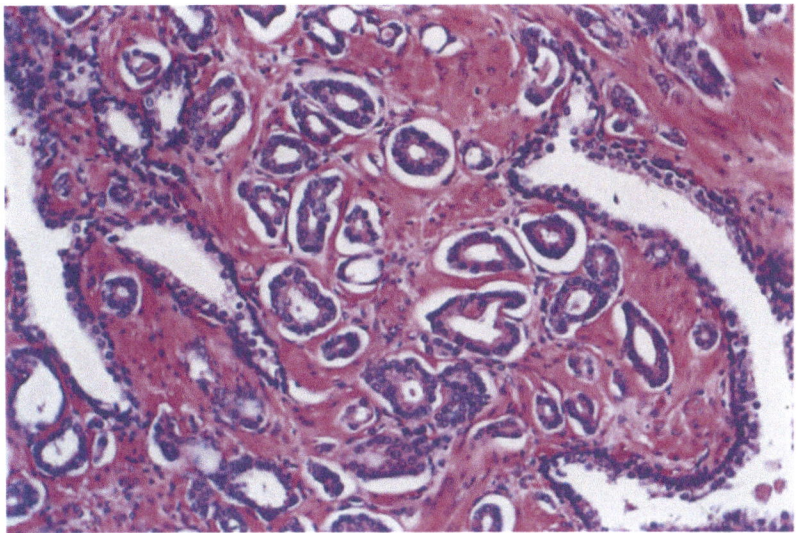

Fig. 10. Adenocarcinoma with abnormal glandular contours and invasive dispersion. Retraction artefact accentuates abnormal contours

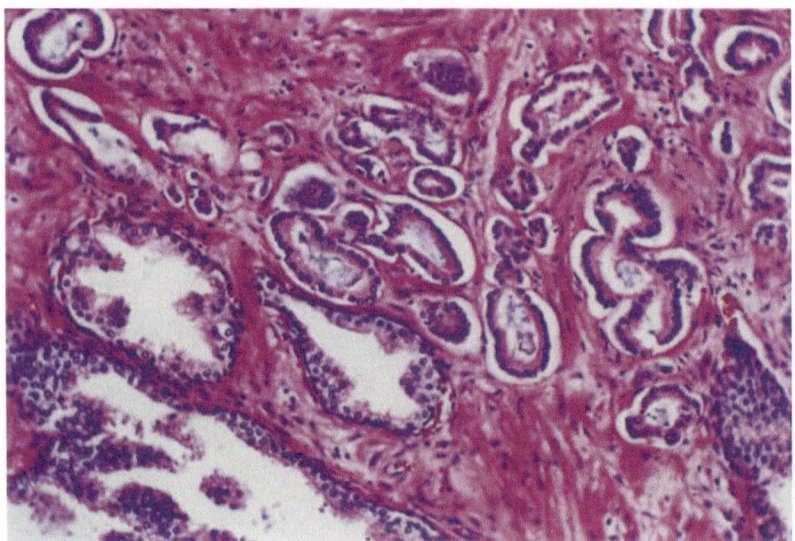

Fig. 11. Adenocarcinoma with intraluminal mucin

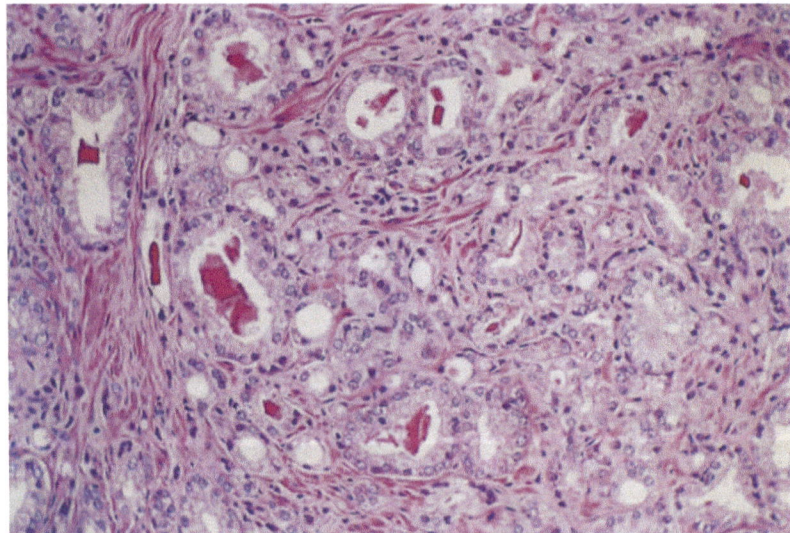

Fig. 12. Adenocarcinoma with crystalloids

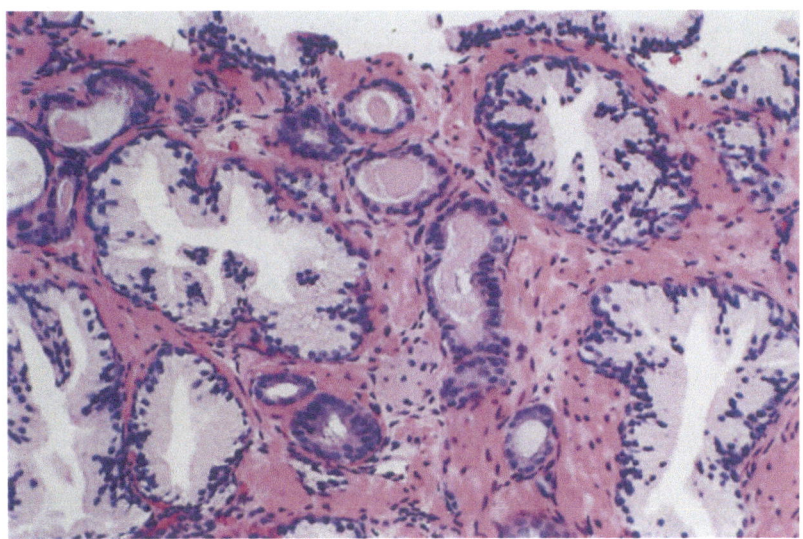

Fig. 13. Adenocarcinoma with invasion around and between benign glands

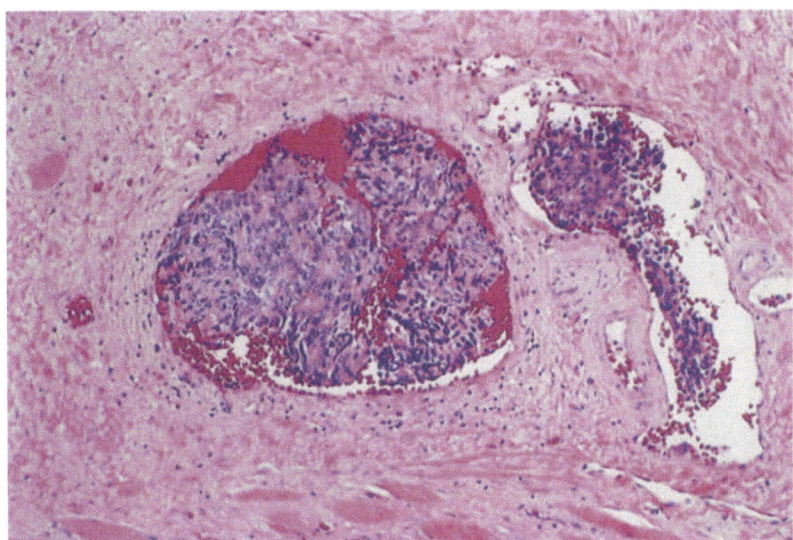

Fig. 14. Adenocarcinoma with vascular invasion

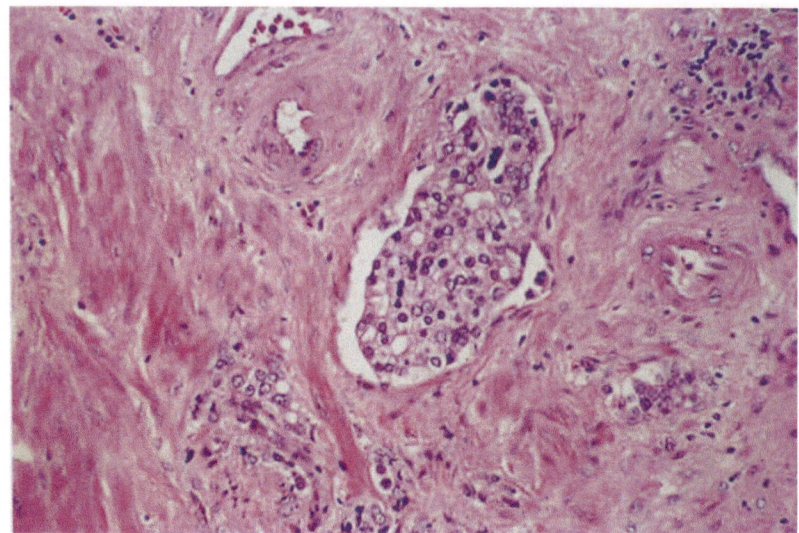

Fig. 15. Adenocarcinoma with lymphatic invasion

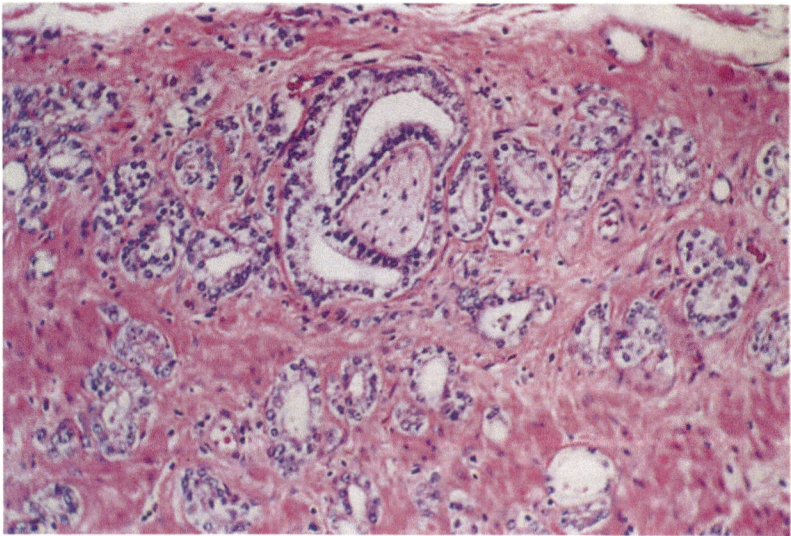

Fig. 16. Adenocarcinoma with perineural space invasion

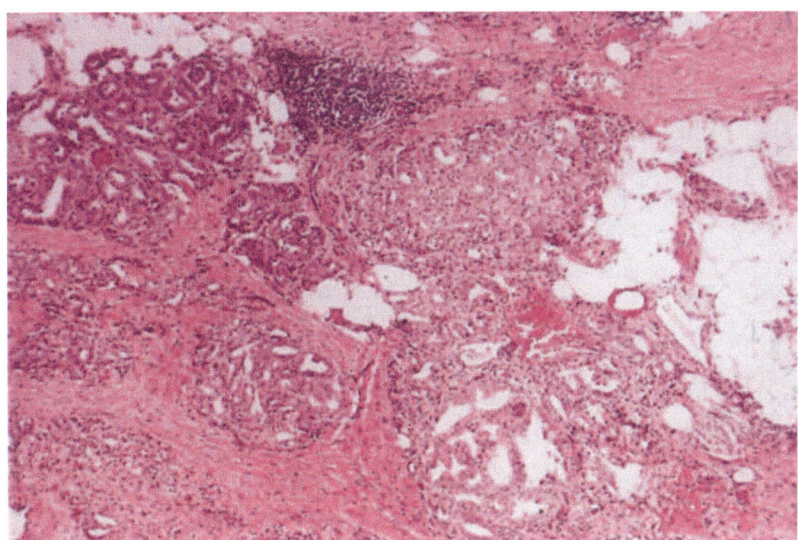

Fig. 17. Adenocarcinoma invading periprostatic adipose tissue

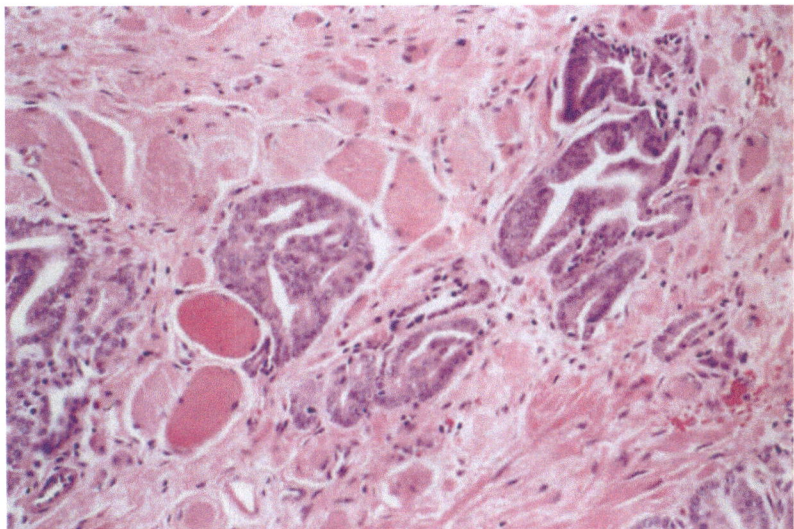

Fig. 18. Adenocarcinoma located in skeletal muscle

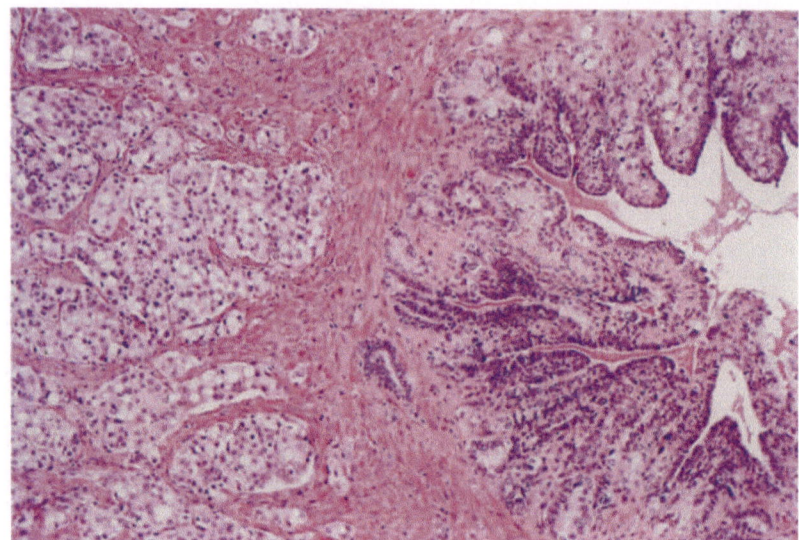

Fig. 19. Adenocarcinoma invading seminal vesicle

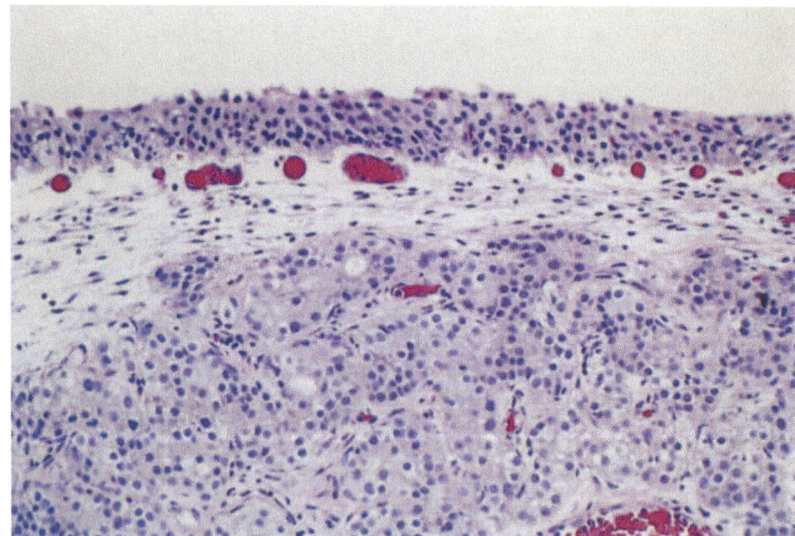

Fig. 20. Adenocarcinoma invading urethral mucosa

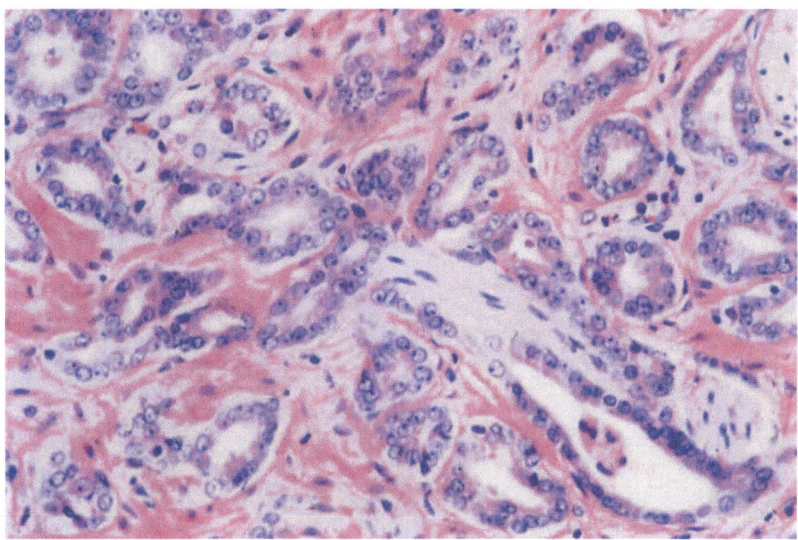

Fig. 21. Adenocarcinoma showing nuclear anaplasia, abnormal glandular morphology and perineural space invasion

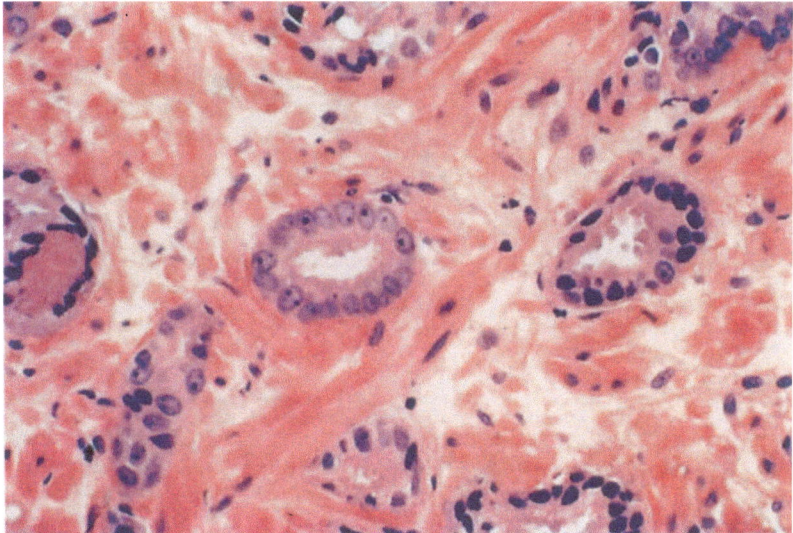

Fig. 22. Adenocarcinoma. The gland in the centre is diagnostic of carcinoma because of the clearly evident nuclear anaplasia

48

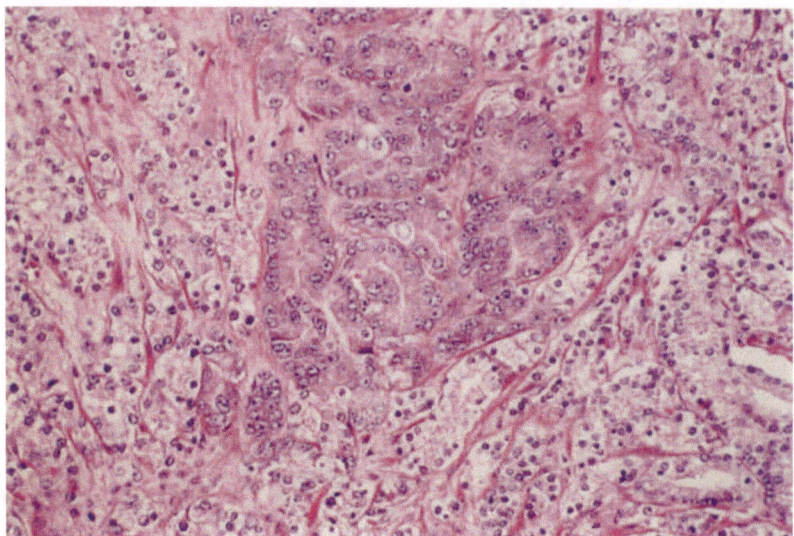

Fig. 23. Adenocarcinoma with both light and dark cells

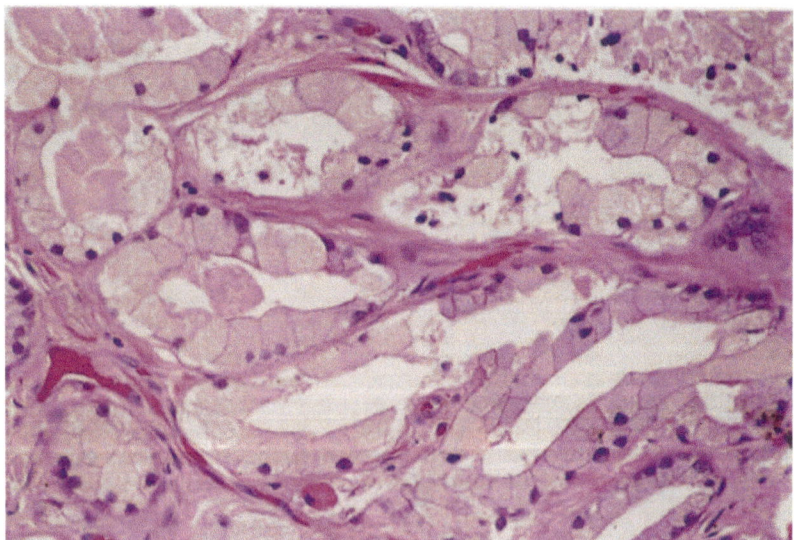

Fig. 24. Adenocarcinoma with foamy cytoplasm

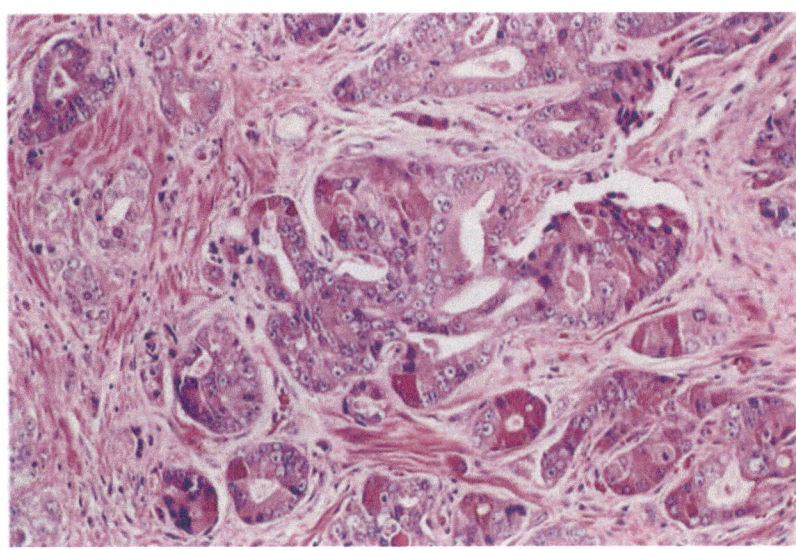

Fig. 25. Adenocarcinoma with endocrine cells

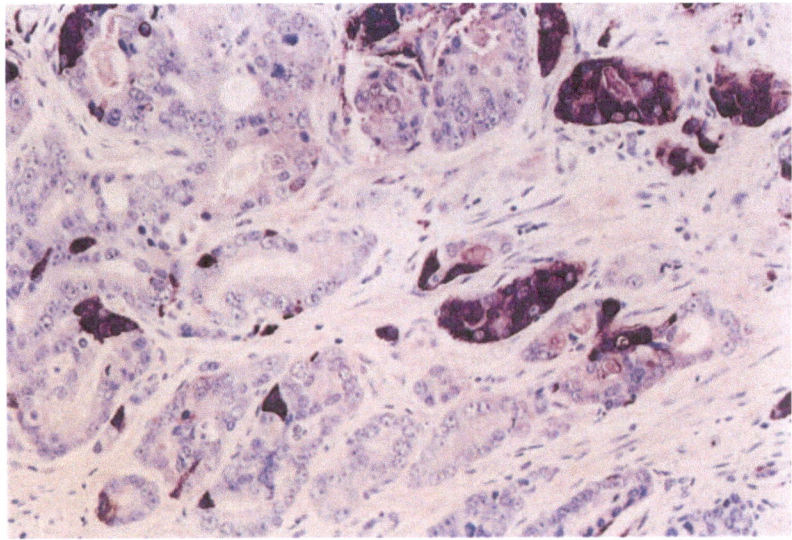

Fig. 26. Adenocarcinoma with antichromogranin. Same field as Fig. 25

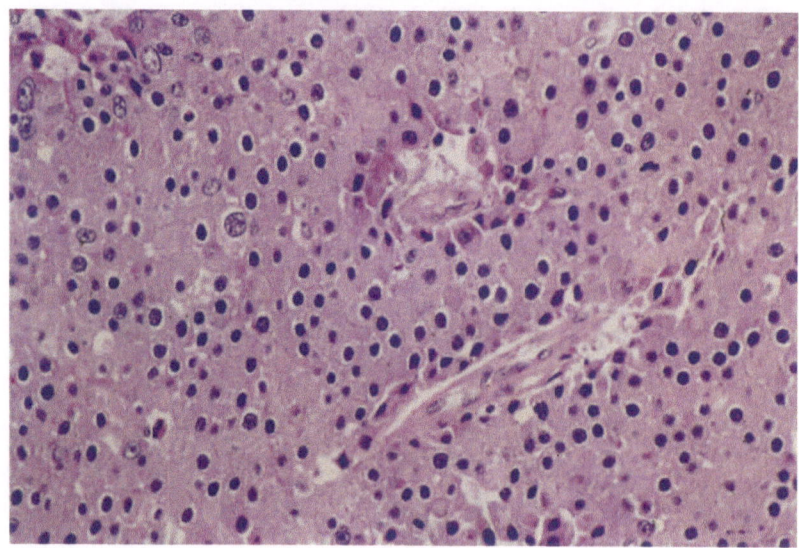

Fig. 27. Adenocarcinoma with oncocytic features

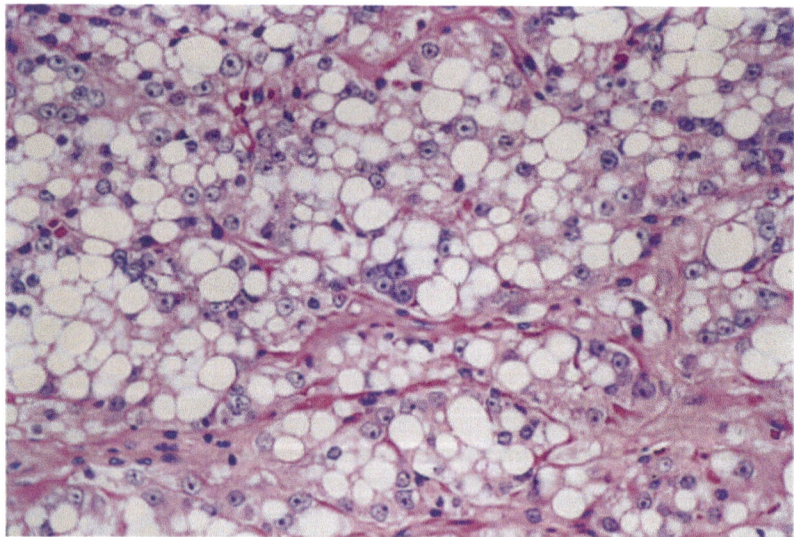

Fig. 28. Adenocarcinoma, vacuolated cell type (mimics signet ring carcinoma)

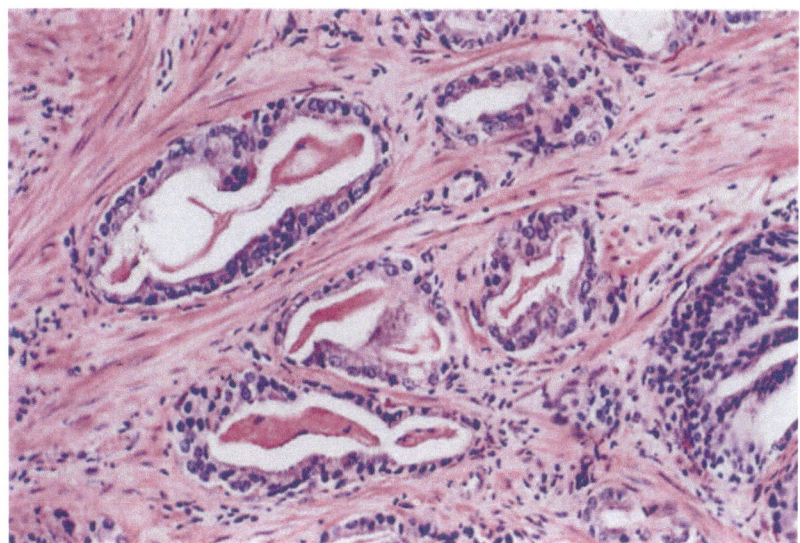

Fig. 29. Adenocarcinoma, well-differentiated

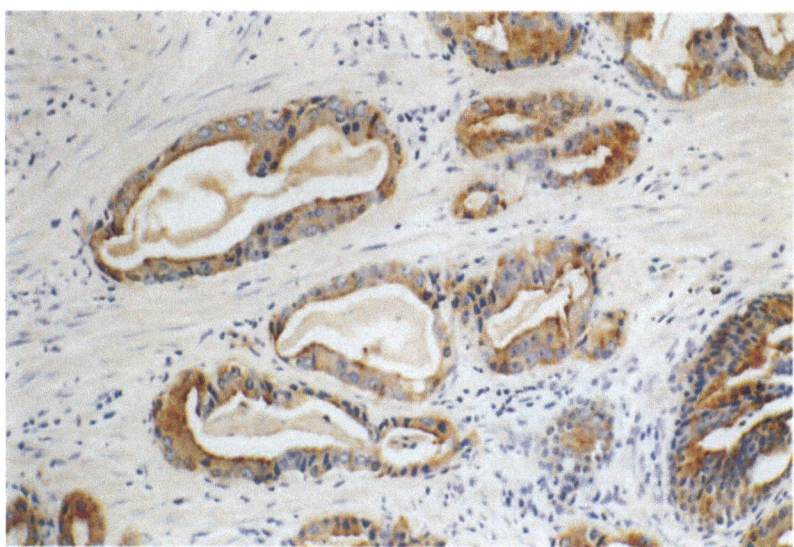

Fig. 30. Adenocarcinoma, anti-PAP. Same field as Fig. 29

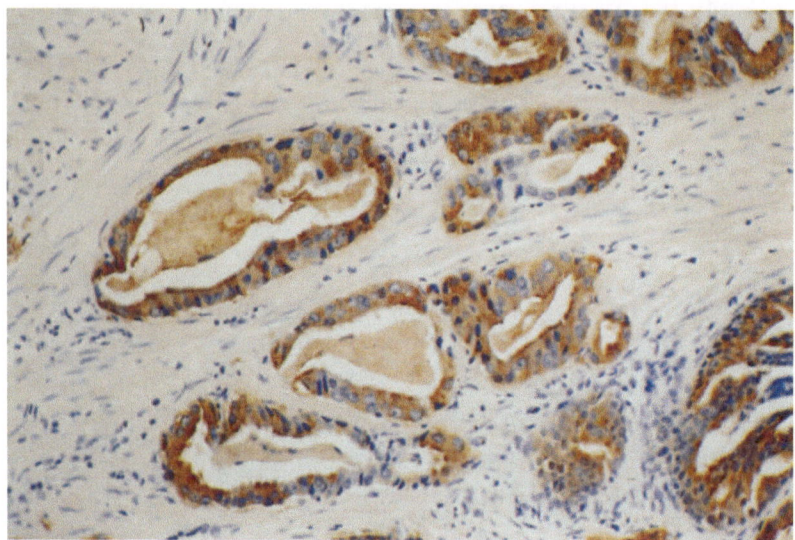

Fig. 31. Adenocarcinoma, anti-PSA. Same field as Fig. 29

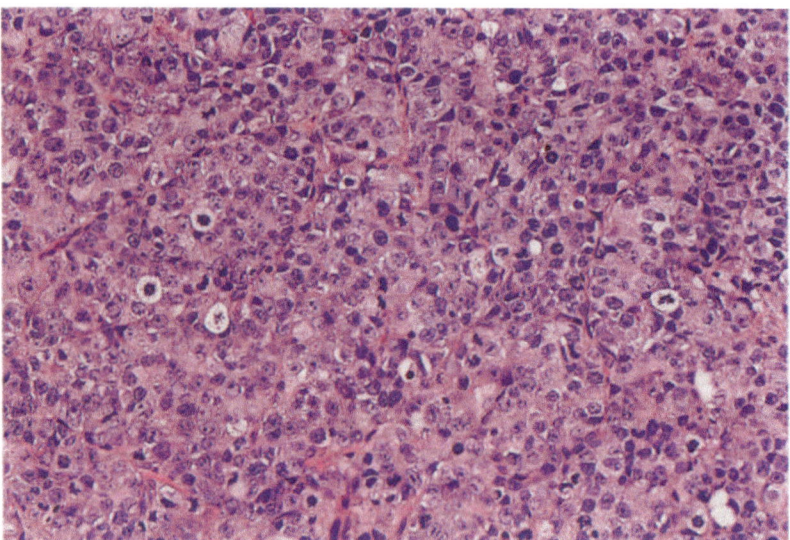

Fig. 32. Adenocarcinoma, poorly differentiated

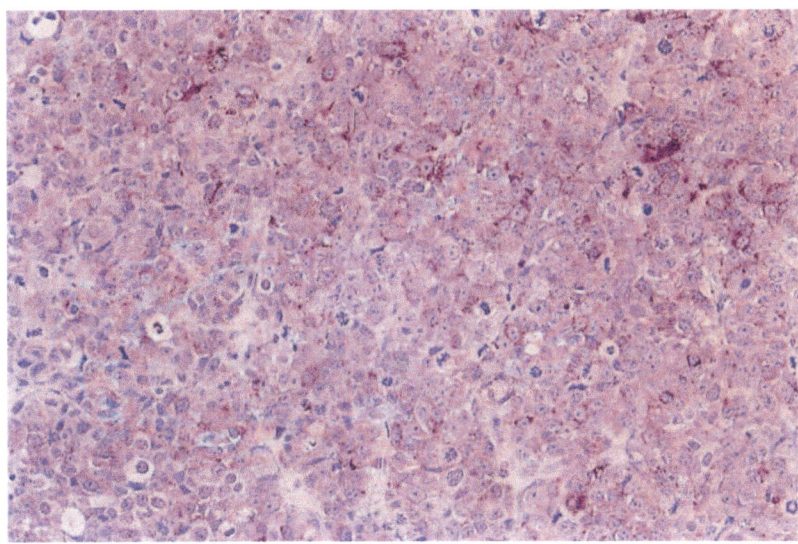

Fig. 33. Adenocarcinoma, anti-PAP. Same field as Fig. 32

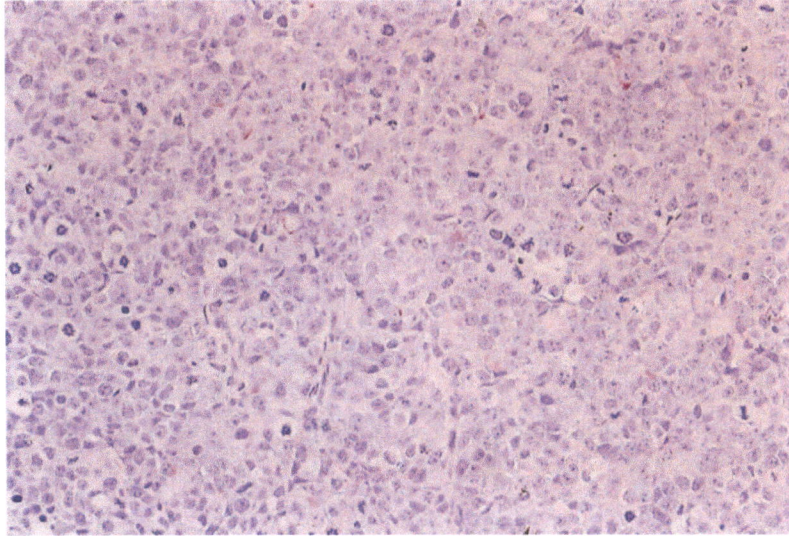

Fig. 34. Adenocarcinoma, anti-PSA. Same field as Fig. 32

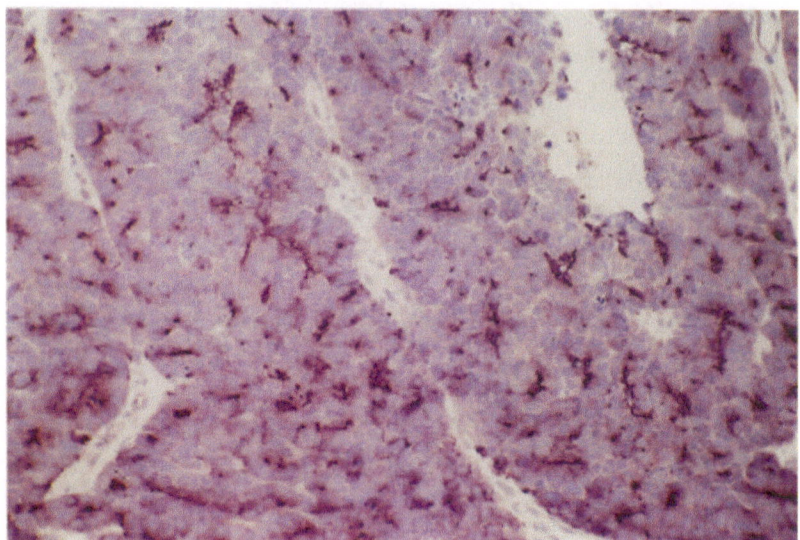

Fig. 35. Adenocarcinoma, anti-PSMA

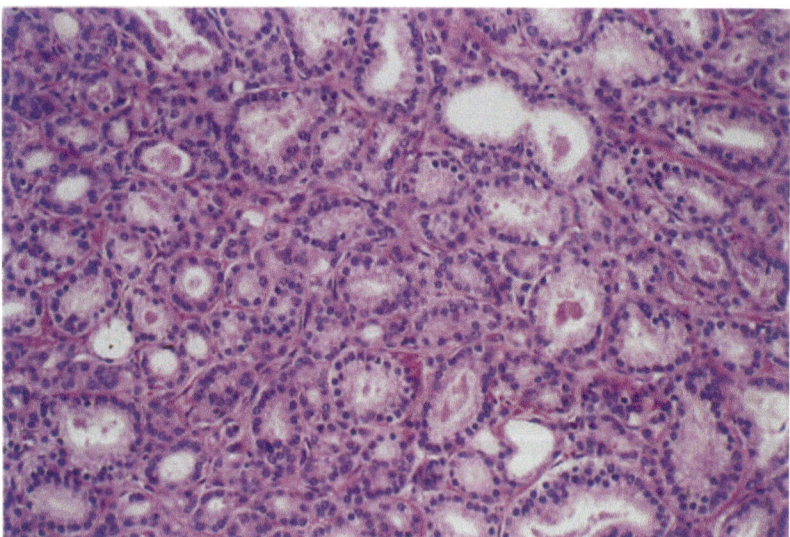

Fig. 36. Adenocarcinoma, small acinar type

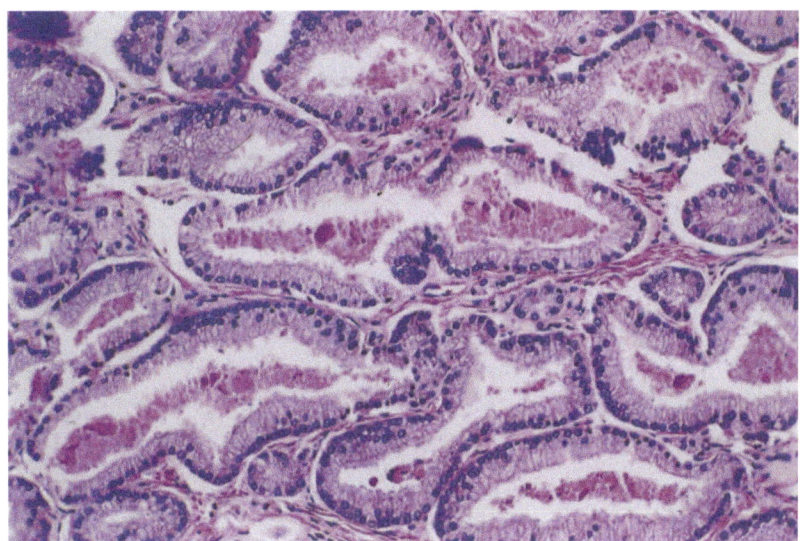

Fig. 37. Adenocarcinoma, large acinar type

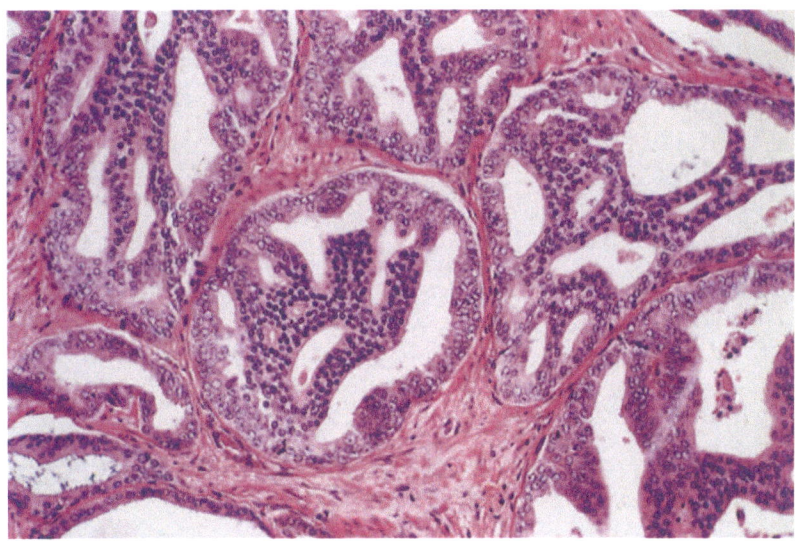

Fig. 38. Adenocarcinoma, cribriform type

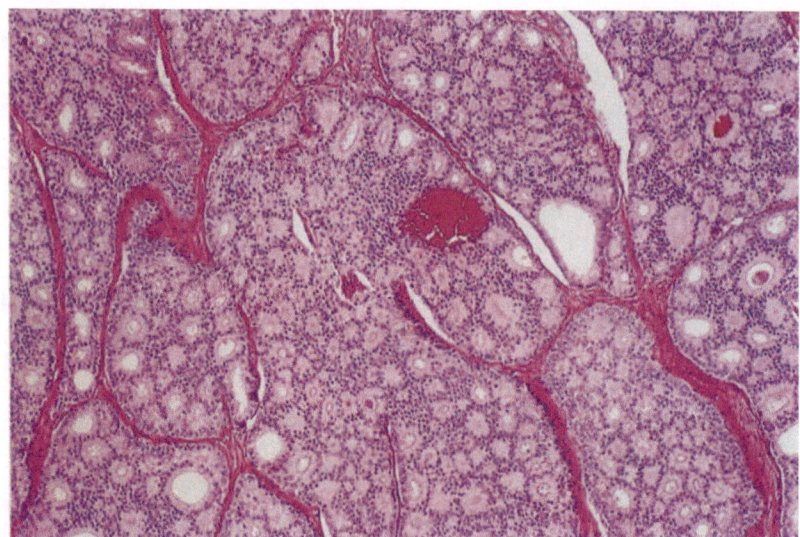

Fig. 39. Adenocarcinoma, fused gland type

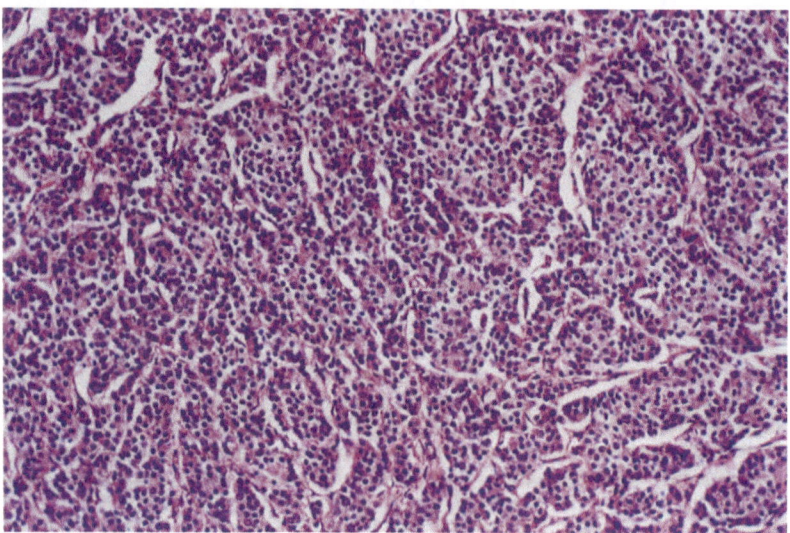

Fig. 40. Adenocarcinoma, poorly differentiated

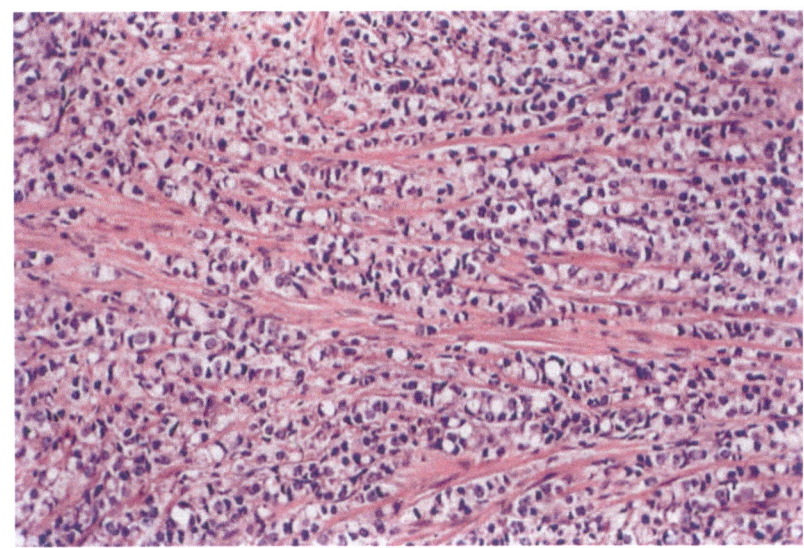

Fig. 41. Adenocarcinoma, poorly differentiated

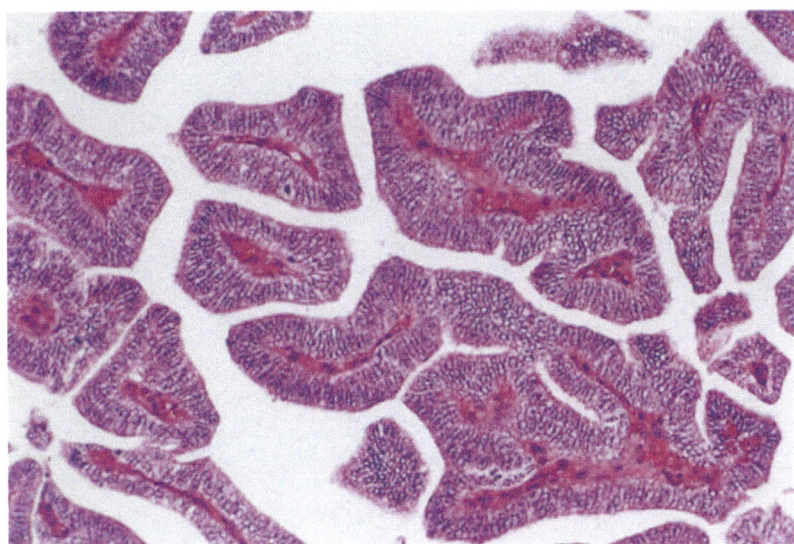

Fig. 42. Adenocarcinoma, papillary type

58

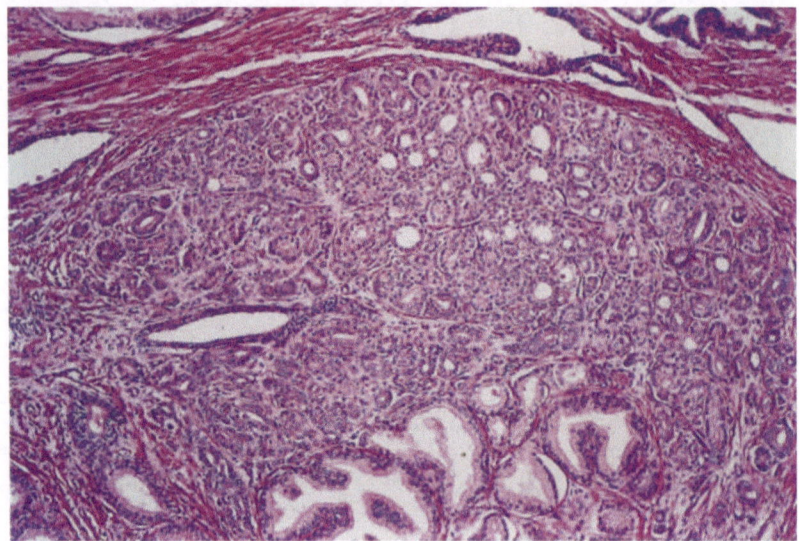

Fig. 43. Adenocarcinoma, Gleason pattern 1 (WHO I+1=2)

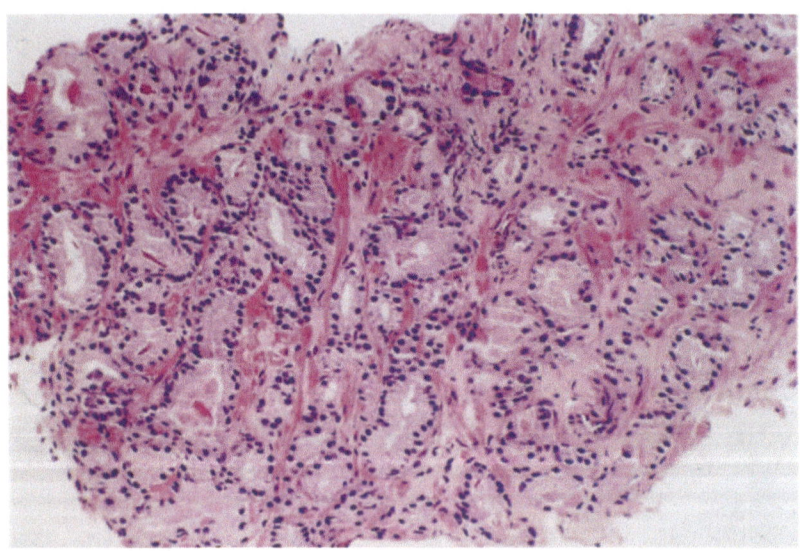

Fig. 44. Adenocarcinoma, Gleason pattern 2 (WHO I+1=2)

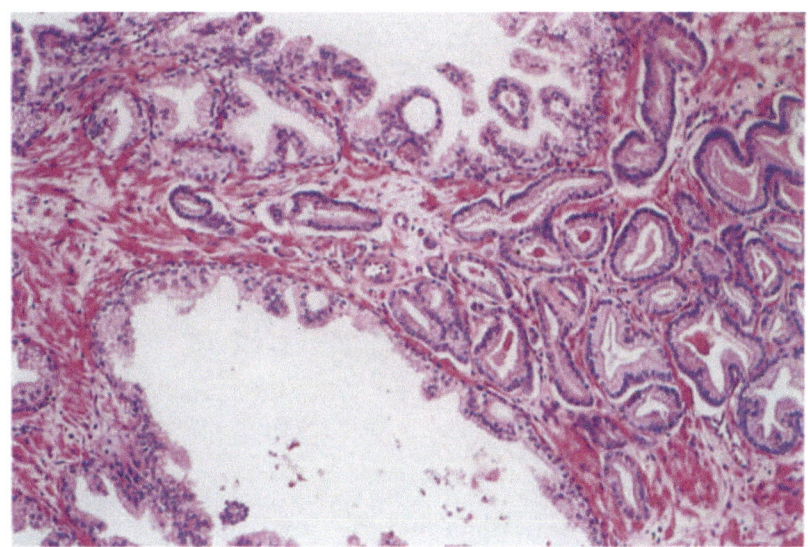

Fig. 45. Adenocarcinoma, Gleason pattern 3 (WHO I+1=2)

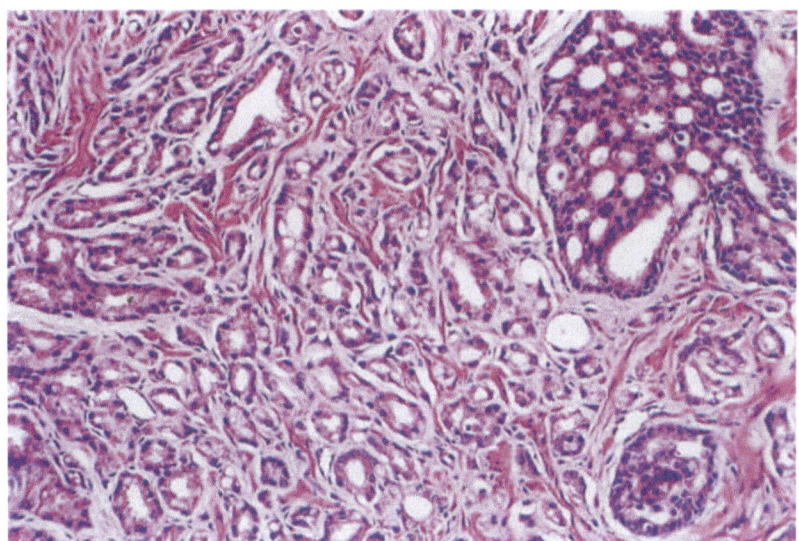

Fig. 46. Adenocarcinoma, Gleason pattern 3 and 4 (WHO I+3=4)

60

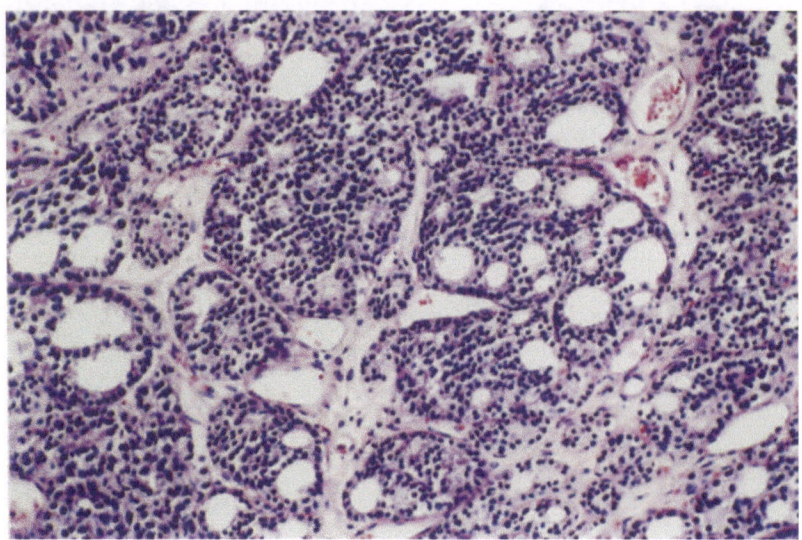

Fig. 47. Adenocarcinoma, Gleason pattern 4 (WHO I+5=6)

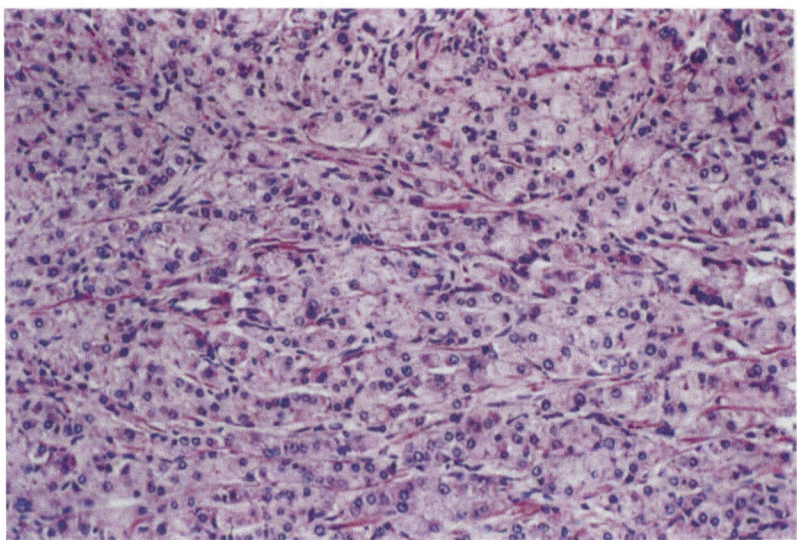

Fig. 48. Adenocarcinoma, Gleason pattern 4 (WHO II+5=7)

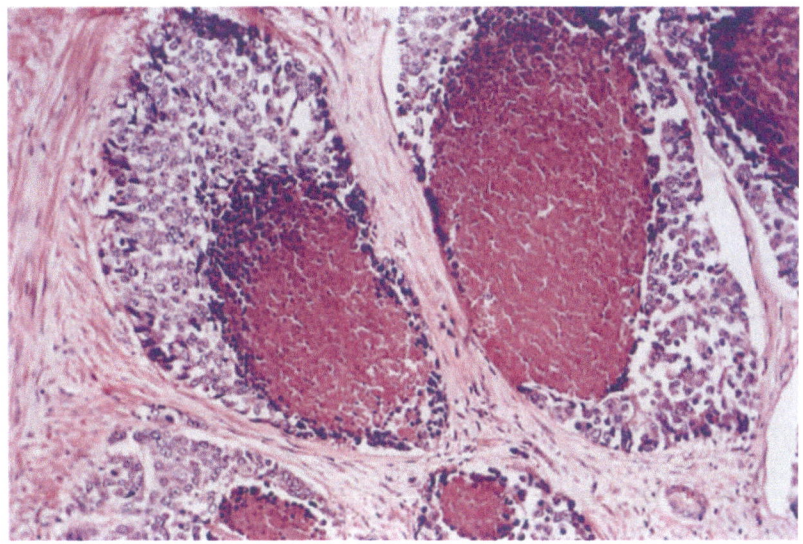

Fig. 49. Adenocarcinoma, Gleason pattern 5 (WHO II+5=7)

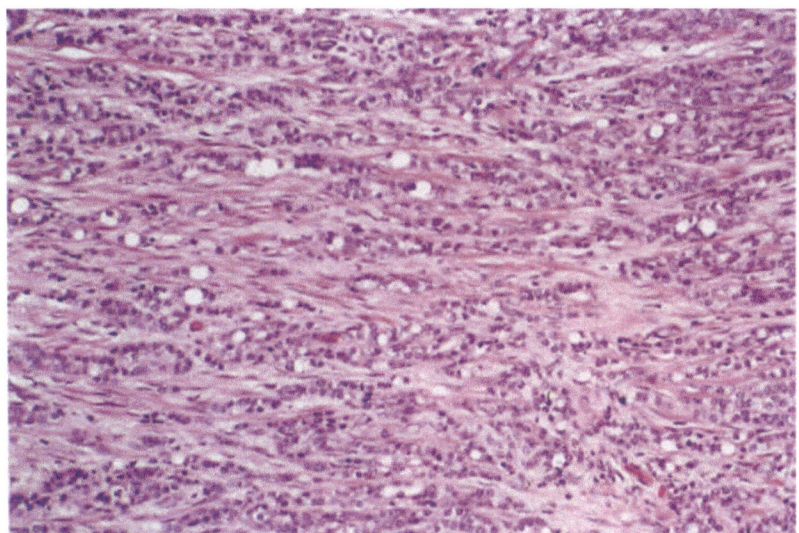

Fig. 50. Adenocarcinoma, Gleason pattern 5 (WHO I+5=6)

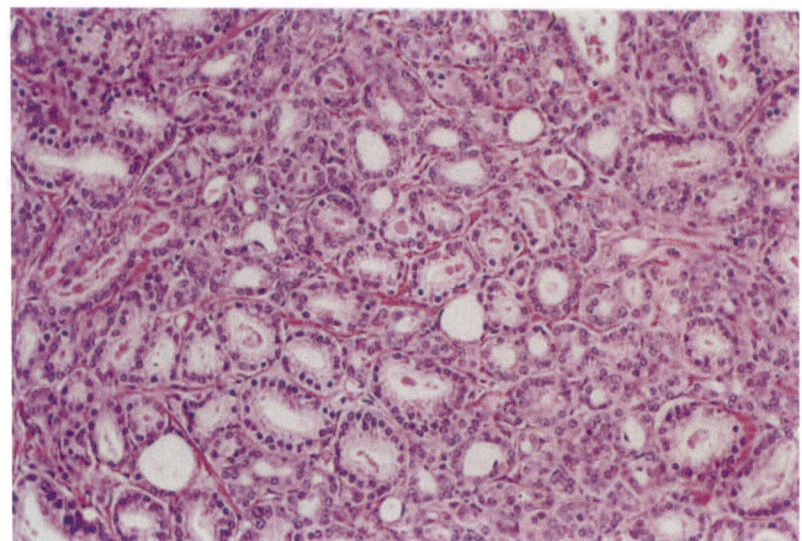

Fig. 51. Adenocarcinoma, nuclear grade I, Gleason pattern 1 (WHO I+1=2)

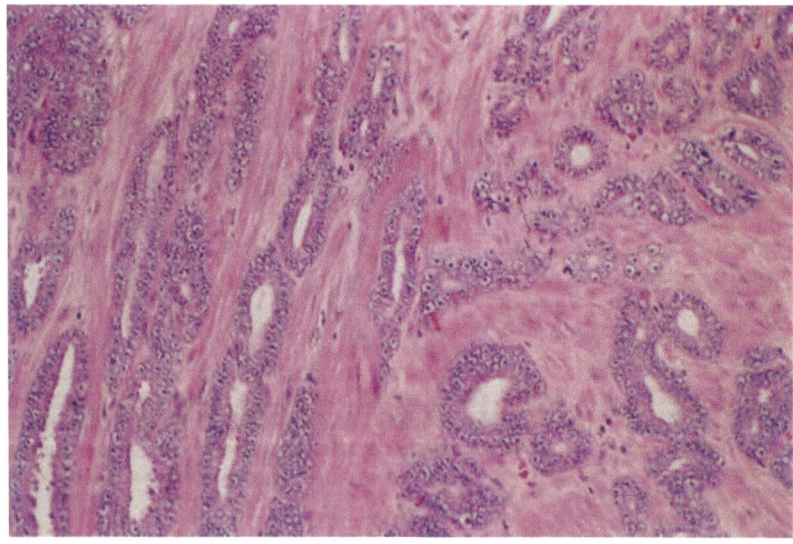

Fig. 52. Adenocarcinoma, nuclear grade II, Gleason pattern 3 (WHO II+1=3)

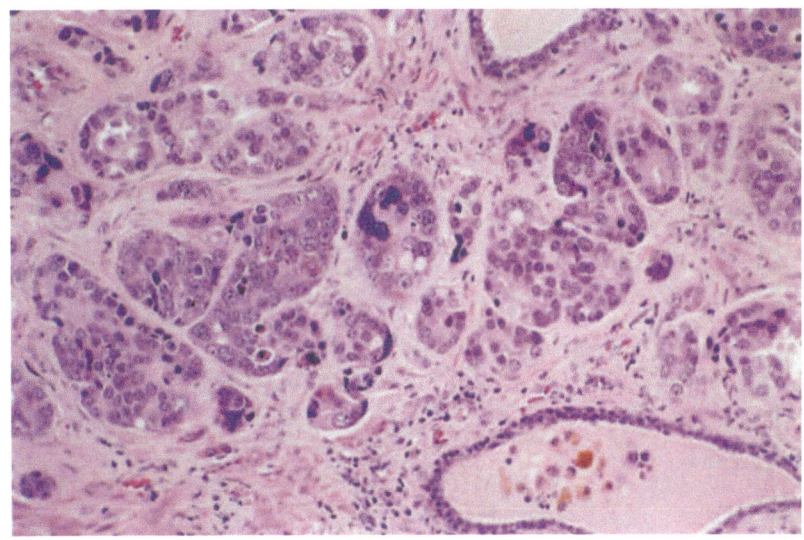

Fig. 53. Adenocarcinoma, nuclear grade III, Gleason pattern 5 (WHO III+5=8)

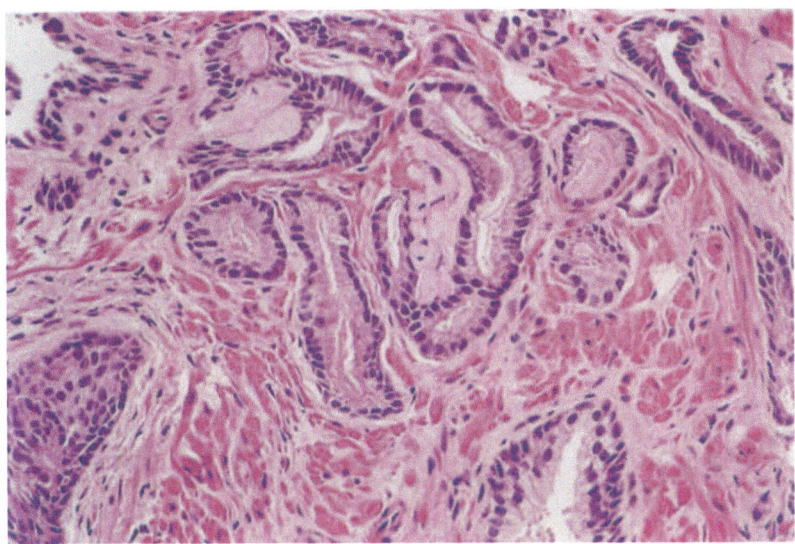

Fig. 54. Adenocarcinoma, well differentiated, Gleason pattern 3 (WHO I+1=2)

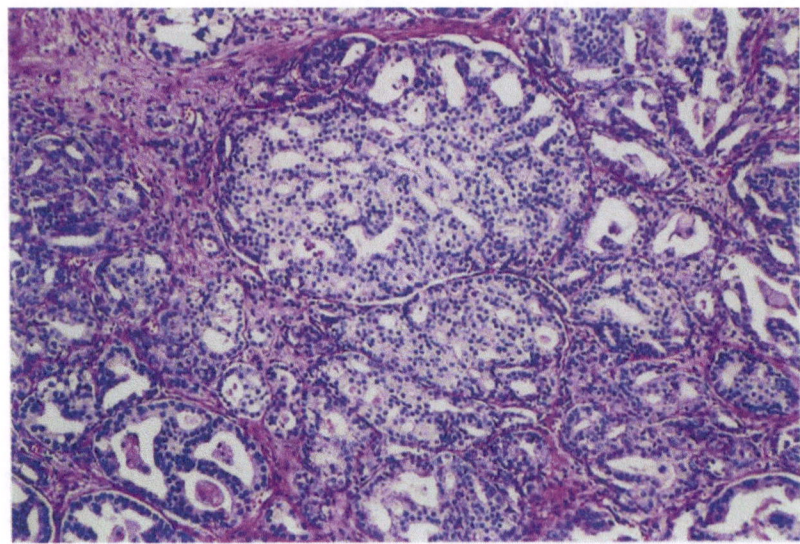

Fig. 55. Adenocarcinoma, moderately differentiated, Gleason pattern 3 and 4 (WHO I+5=6)

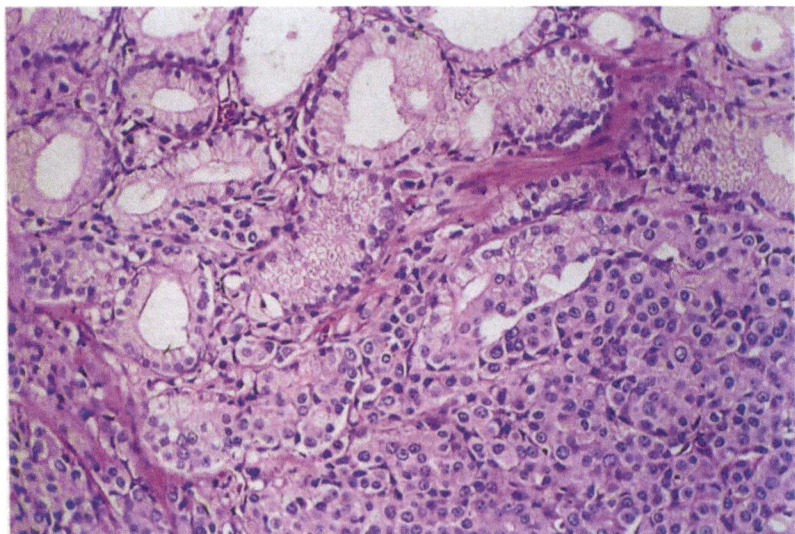

Fig. 56. Adenocarcinoma, well and poorly differentiated, Gleason patterns 2 and 5 (WHO II+5=7)

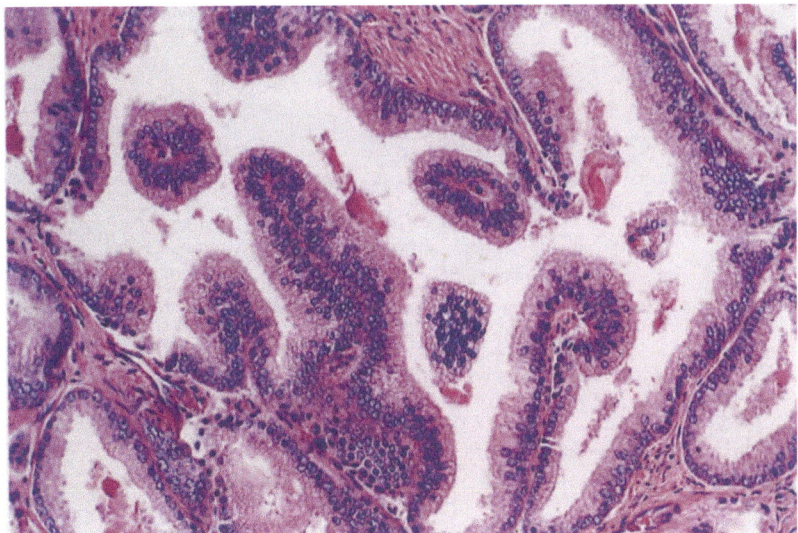

Fig. 57. Adenocarcinoma, pseudohyperplastic type

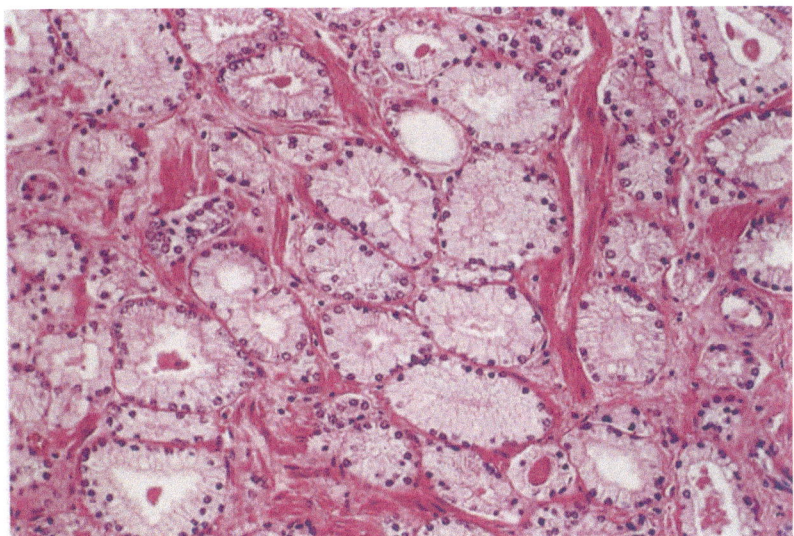

Fig. 58. Adenocarcinoma, pseudohyperplastic type

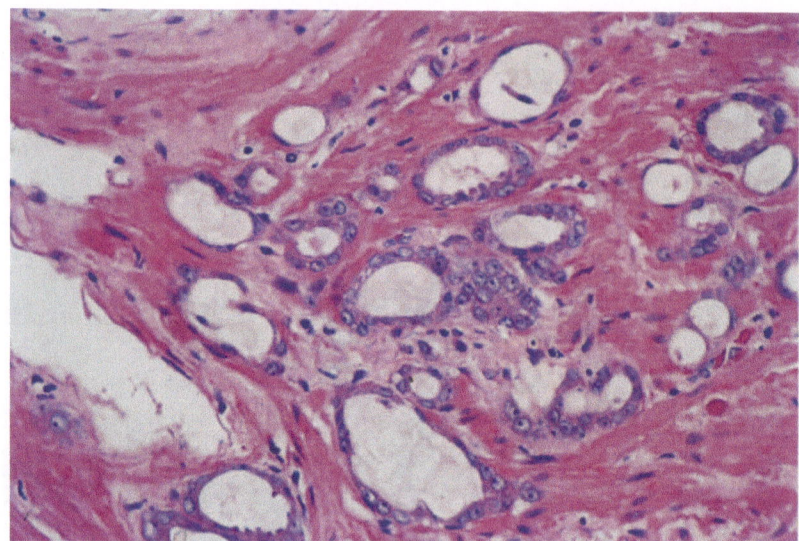

Fig. 59. Adenocarcinoma, atrophy-like

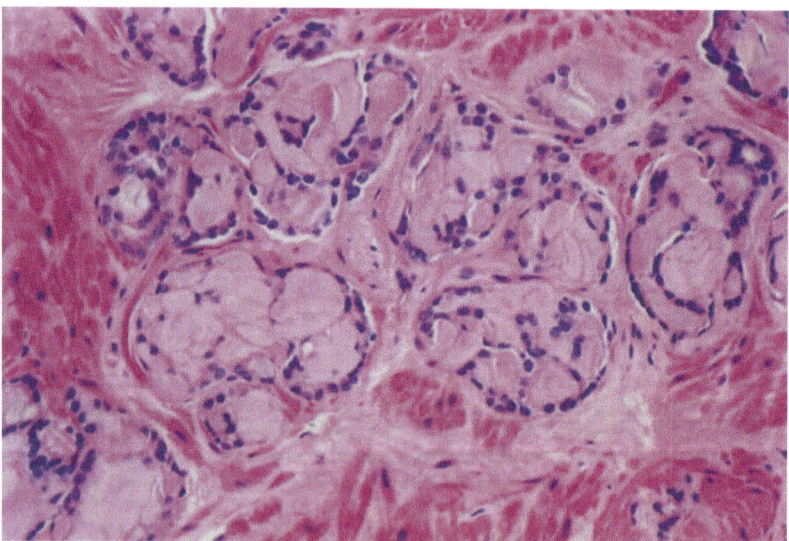

Fig. 60. Adenocarcinoma with hyaline globules

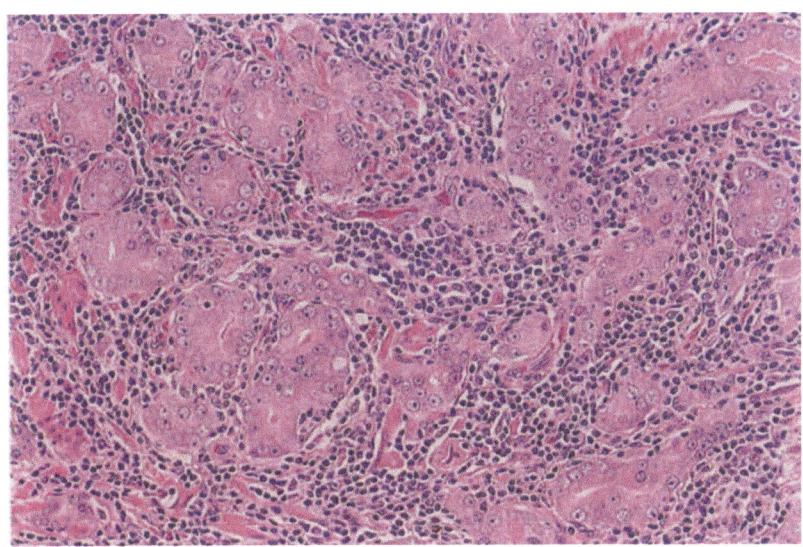

Fig. 61. Adenocarcinoma with lymphocytic infiltrate

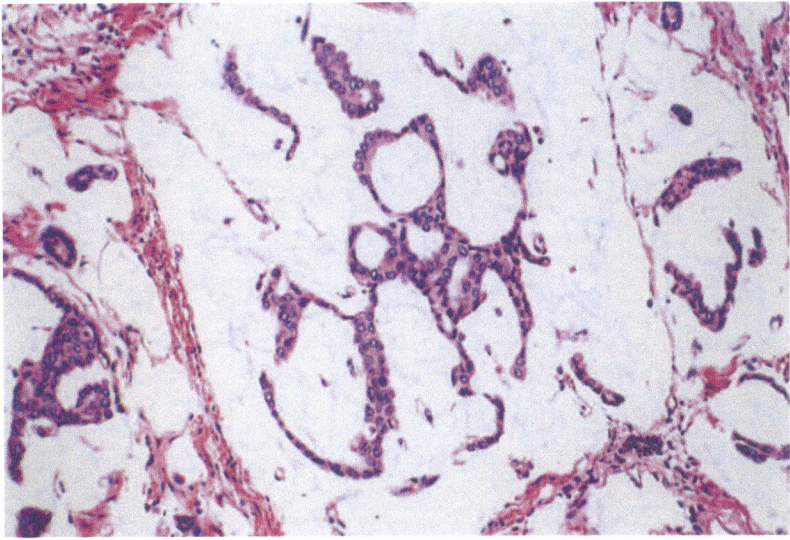

Fig. 62. Adenocarcinoma, mucinous type

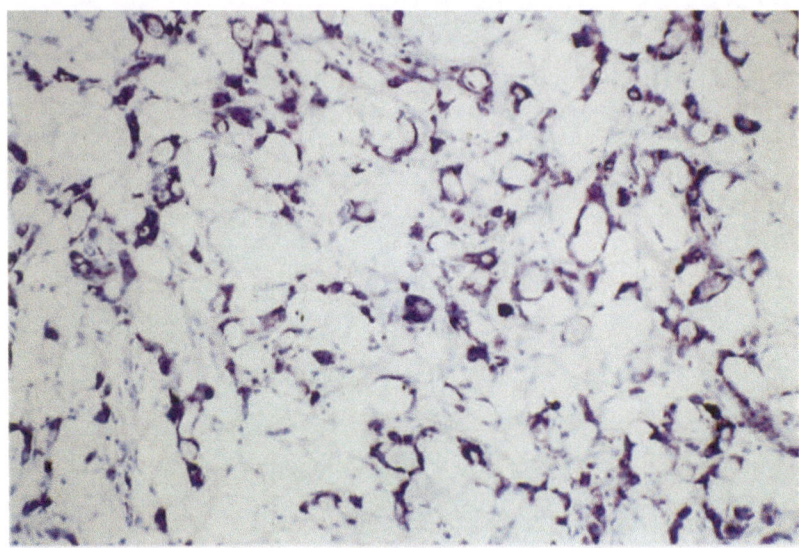

Fig. 63. Adenocarcinoma, mucinous type, anti-PSA

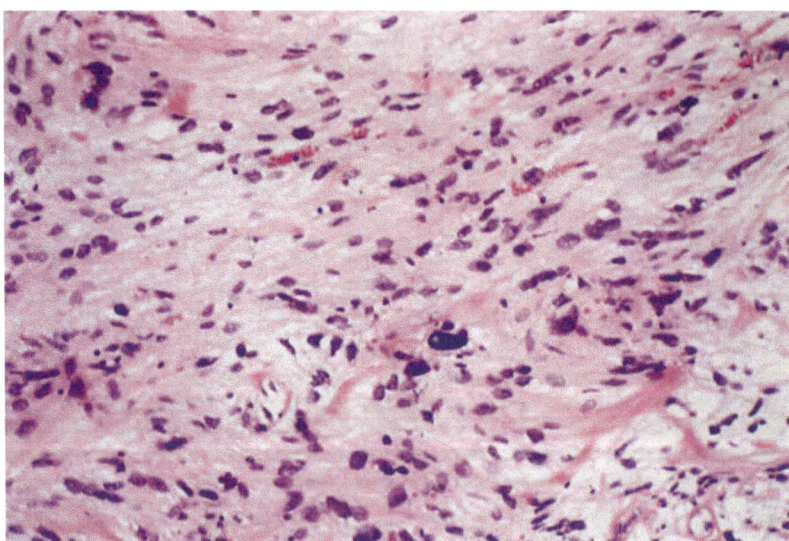

Fig. 64. Spindle cell carcinoma

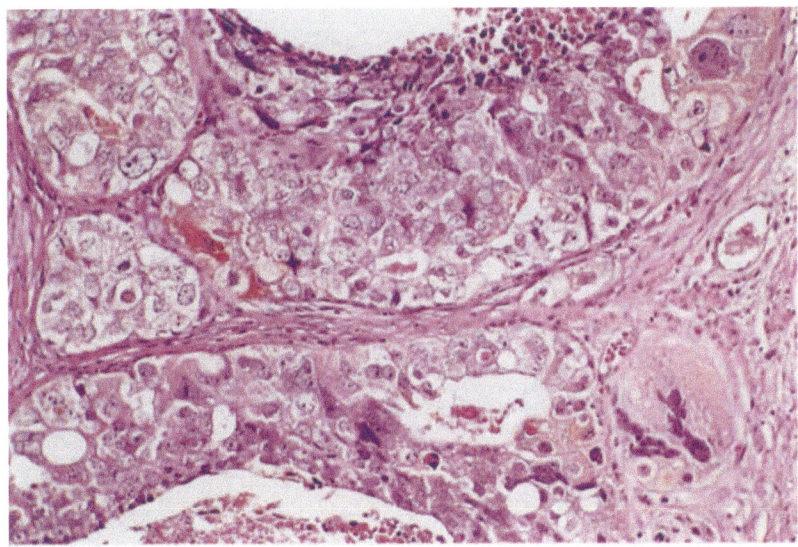

Fig. 65. Adenocarcinoma with marked anaplasia

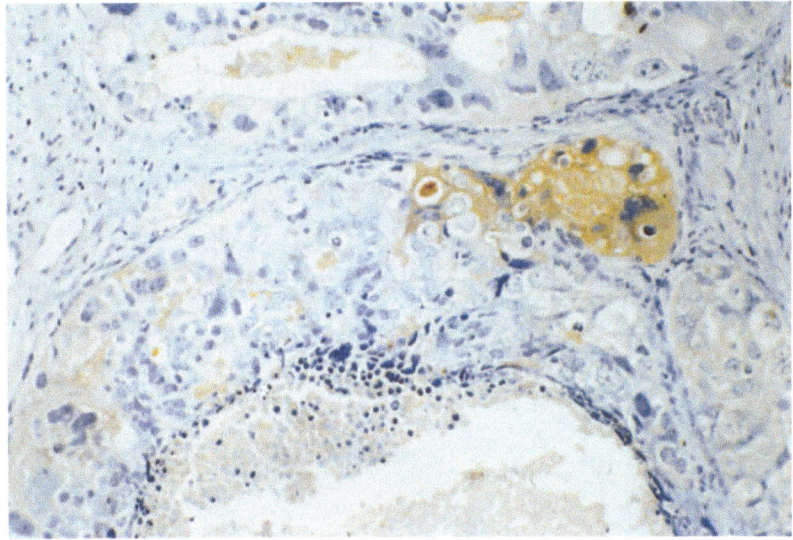

Fig. 66. Adenocarcinoma, anti-HCG. Same field as Fig. 65

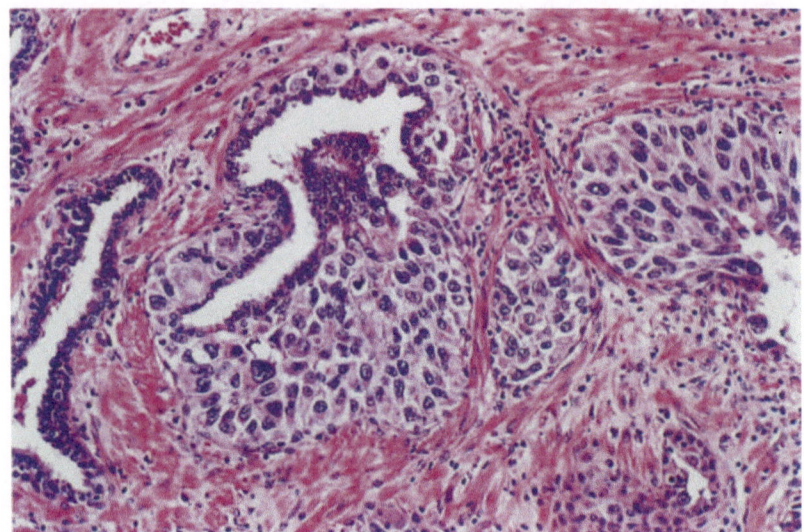

Fig. 67. Urothelial carcinoma, prostatic ducts

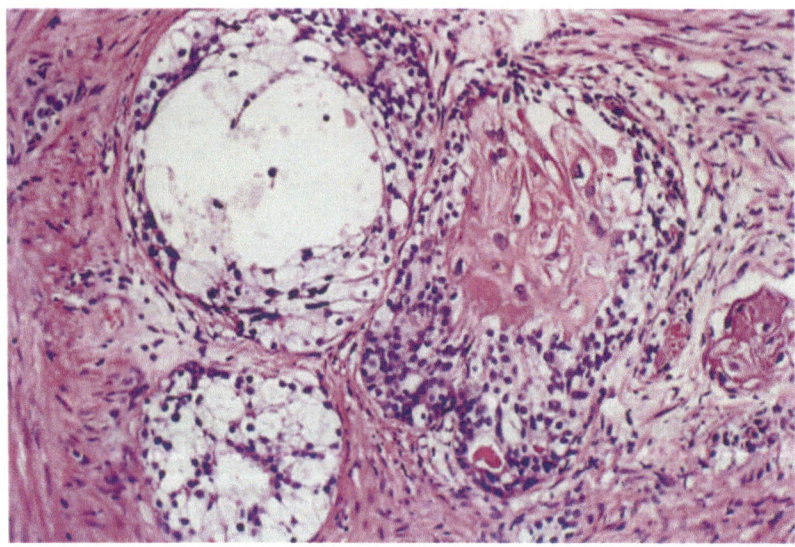

Fig. 68. Squamous cell carcinoma evolving from treated prostatic carcinoma

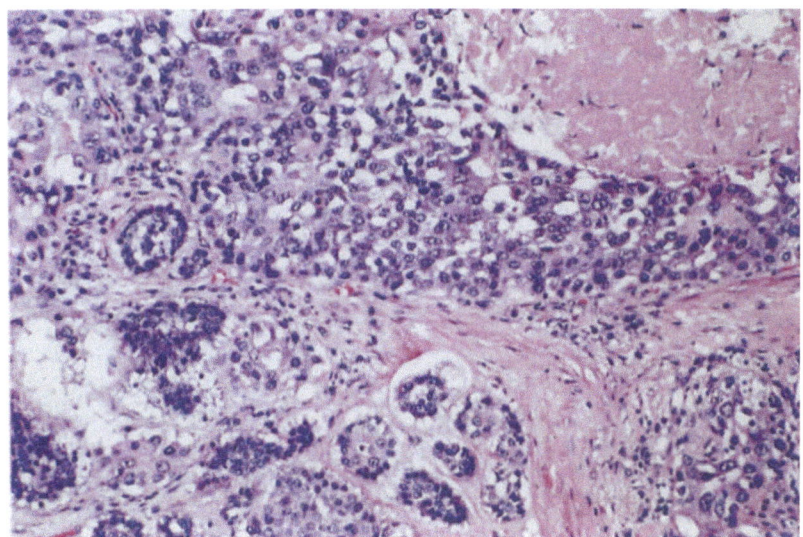

Fig. 69. Basal cell carcinoma

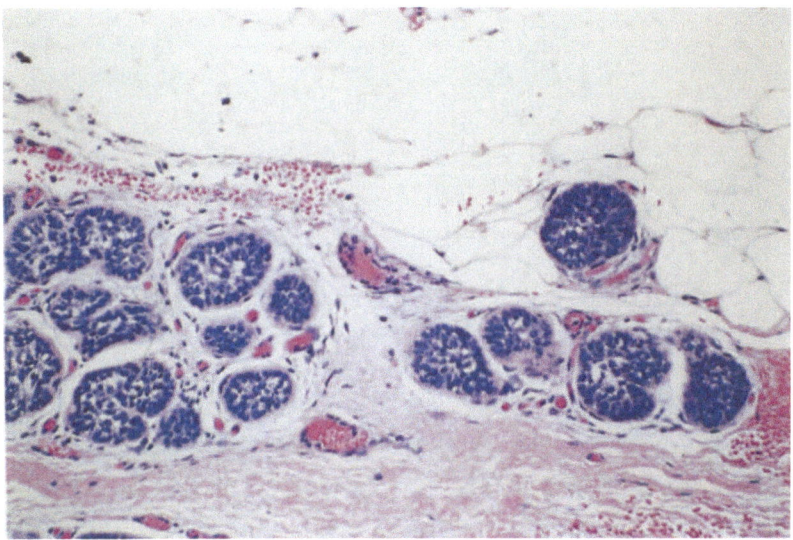

Fig. 70. Basal cell carcinoma invading periprostatic adipose tissue

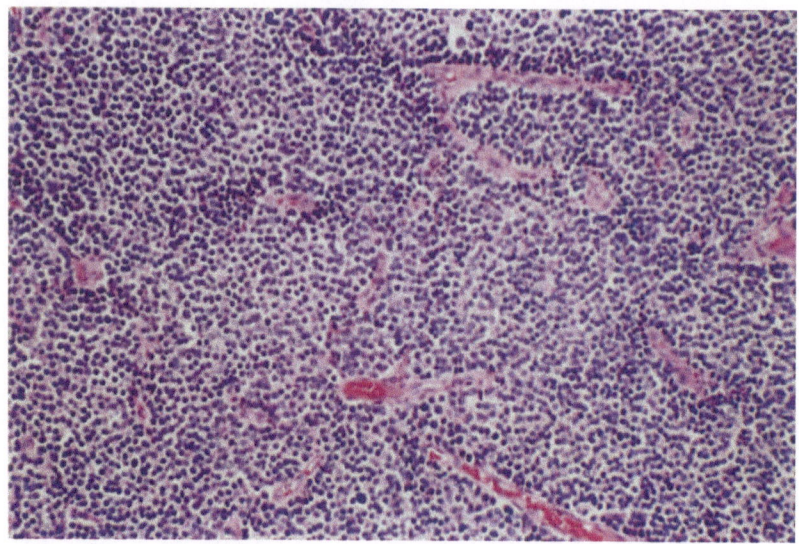

Fig. 71. Small cell carcinoma

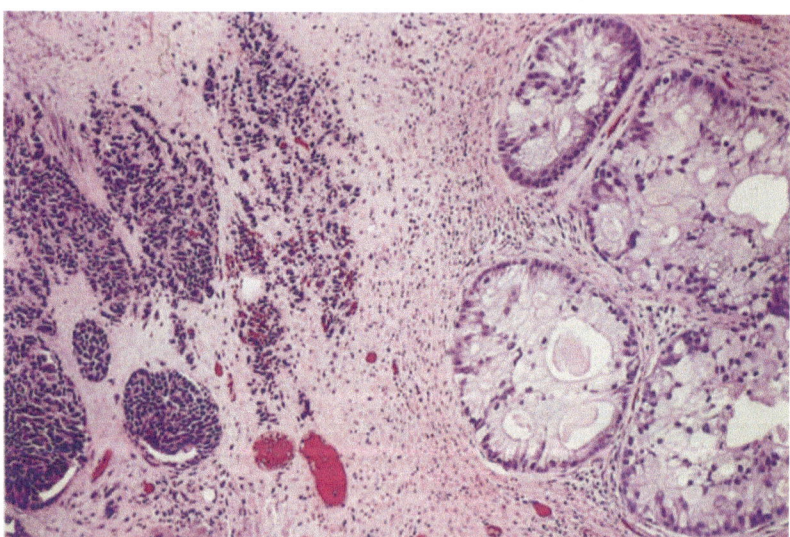

Fig. 72. Prostatic adenocarcinoma with component of small cell carcinoma

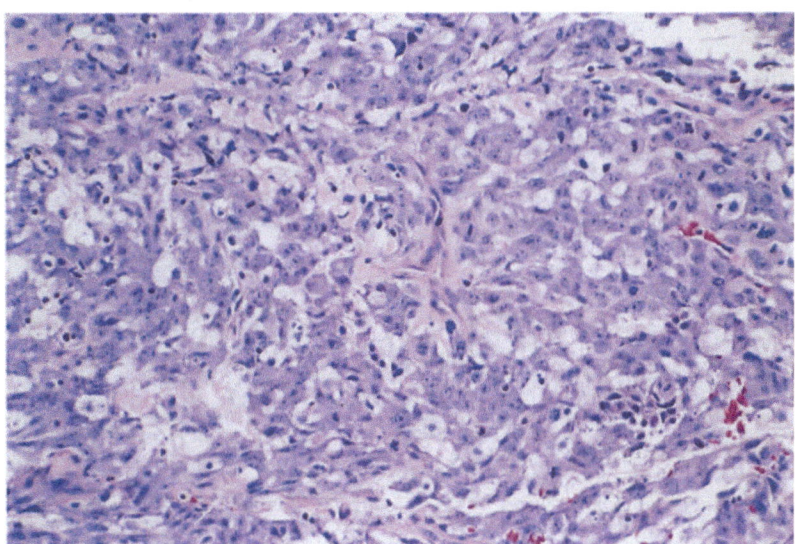

Fig. 73. Undifferentiated carcinoma

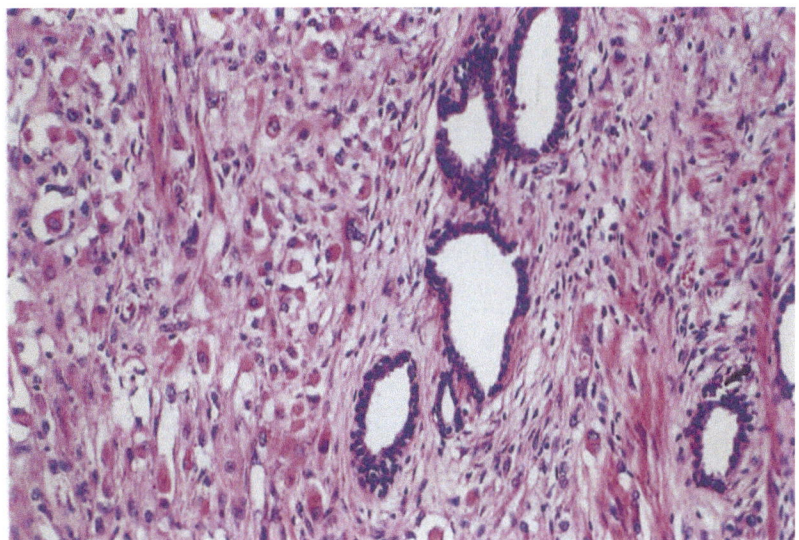

Fig. 74. Rhabdomyosarcoma

74

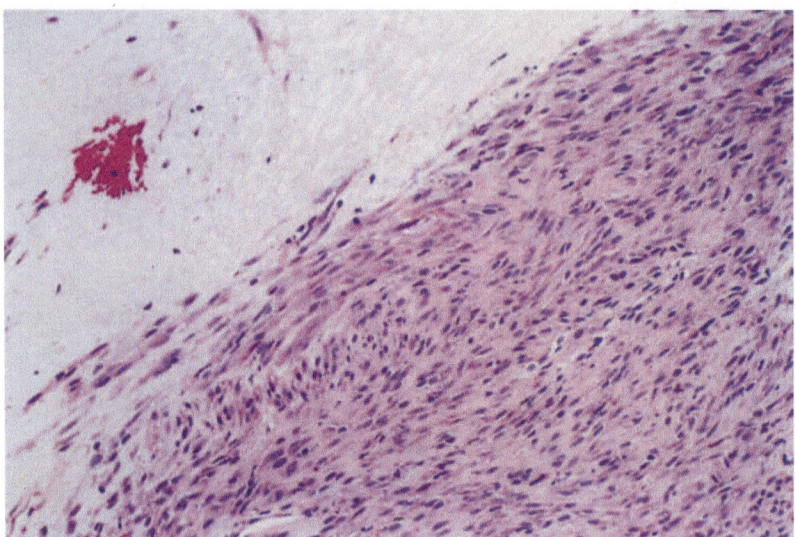

Fig. 75. Leiomyosarcoma

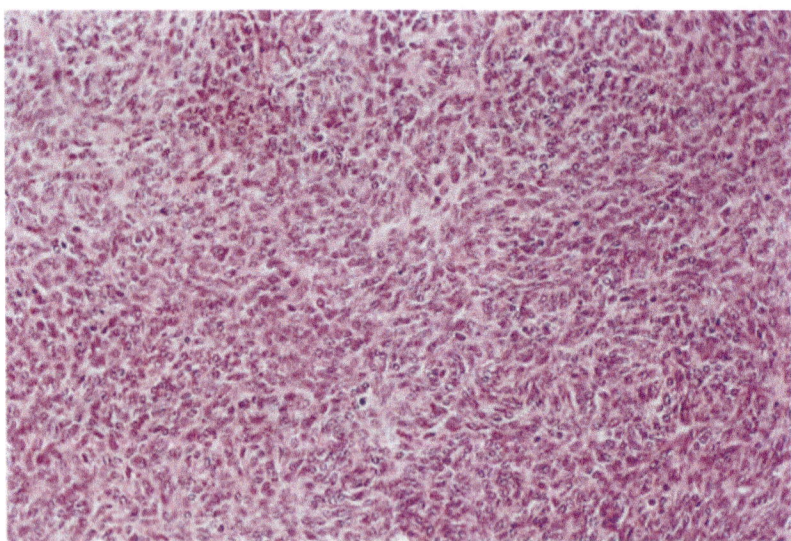

Fig. 76. Prostatic stromal sarcoma

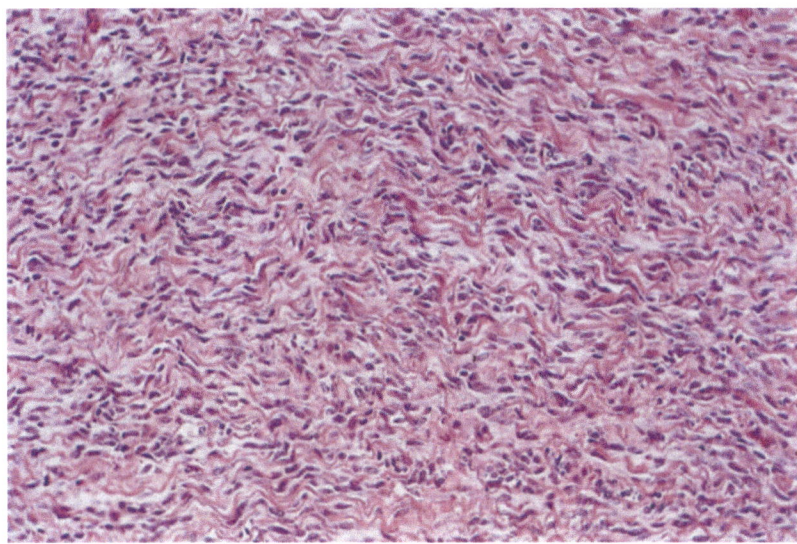

Fig. 77. Prostatic stromal sarcoma with more prominent collagen

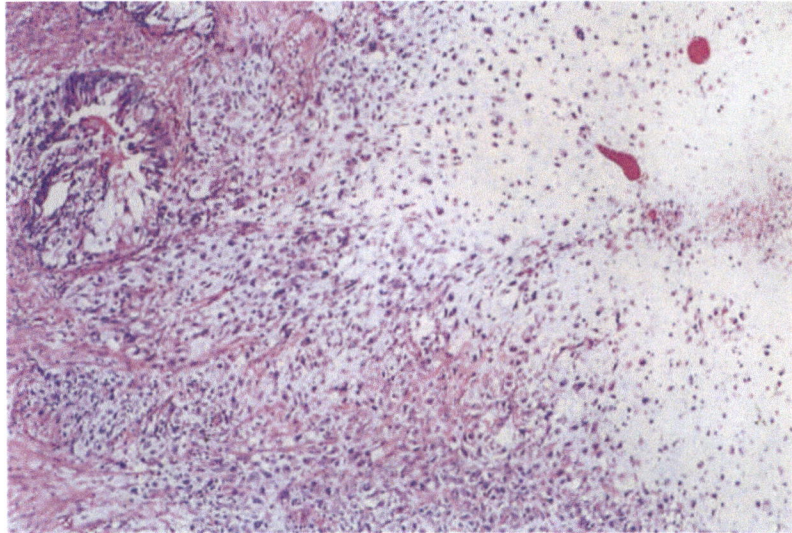

Fig. 78. Carcinosarcoma (adenocarcinoma and chondrosarcoma)

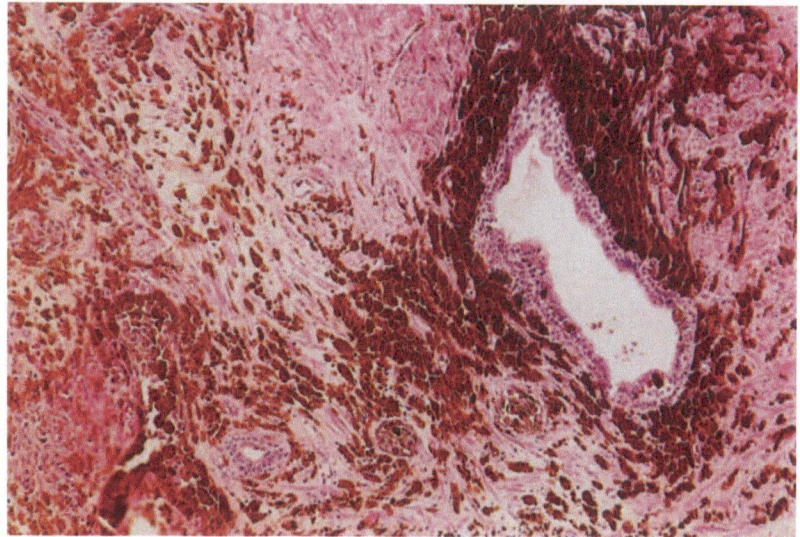

Fig. 79. Melanoma

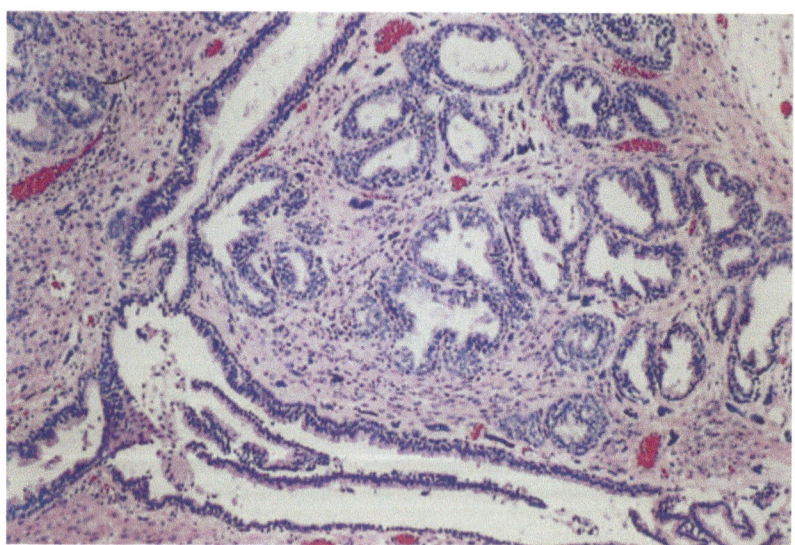

Fig. 80. Phyllodes tumour

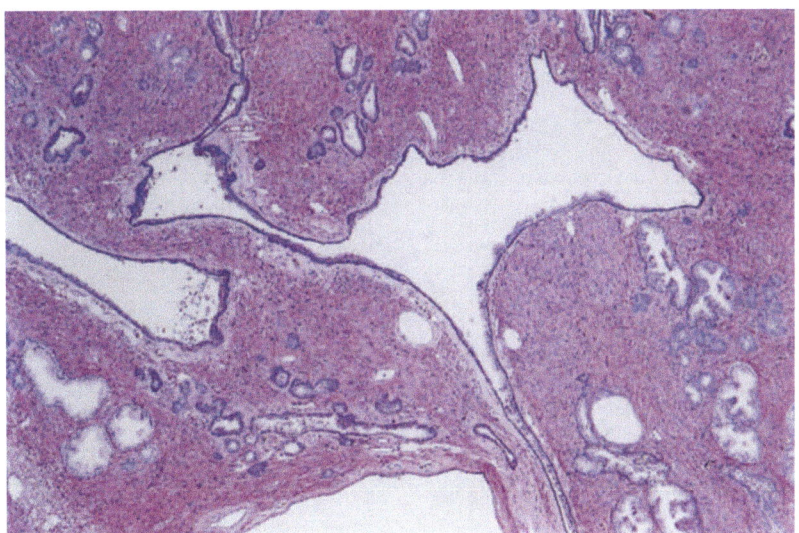

Fig. 81. Phyllodes tumour

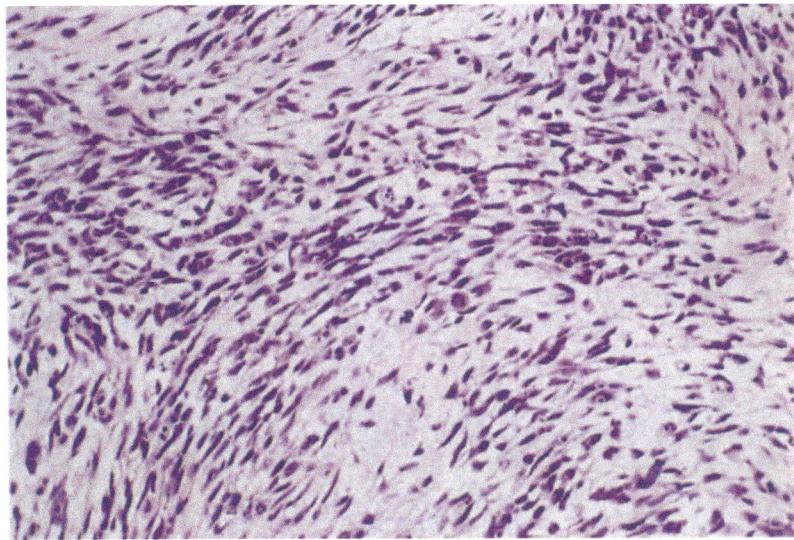

Fig. 82. Malignant phyllodes tumour. Same case as in Fig. 81

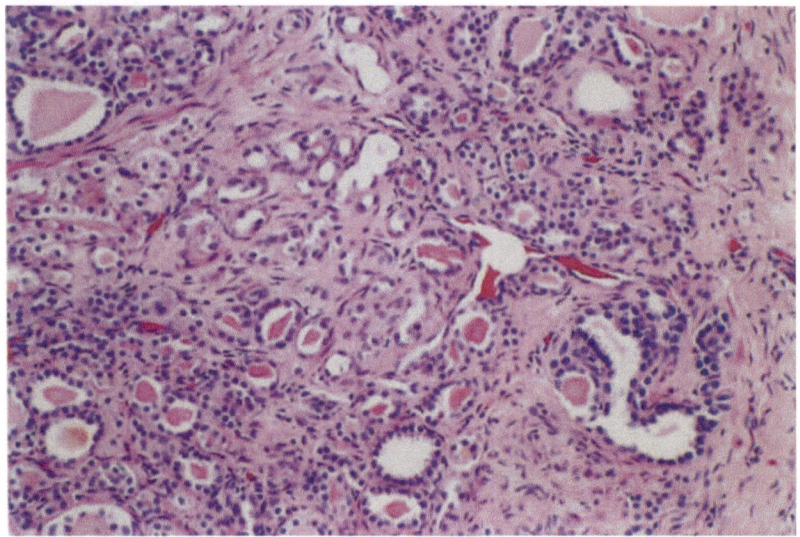

Fig. 83. Mesonephric remnants, hyperplastic

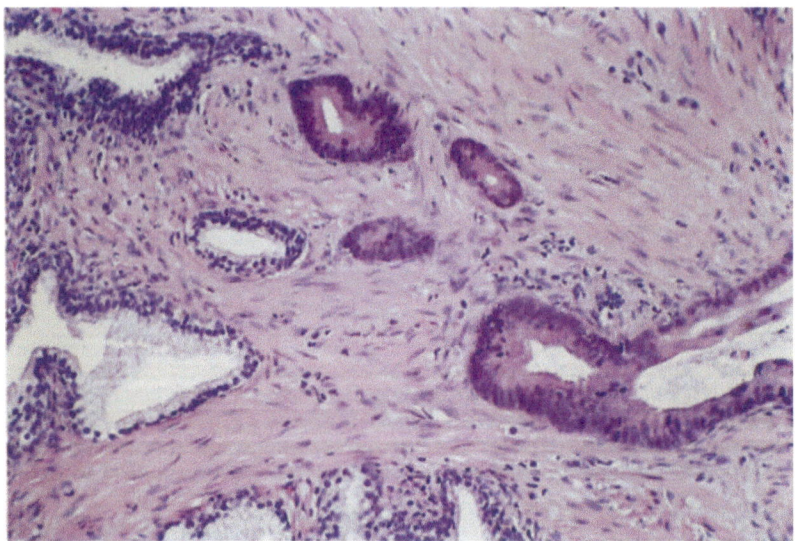

Fig. 84. Metastatic colon carcinoma

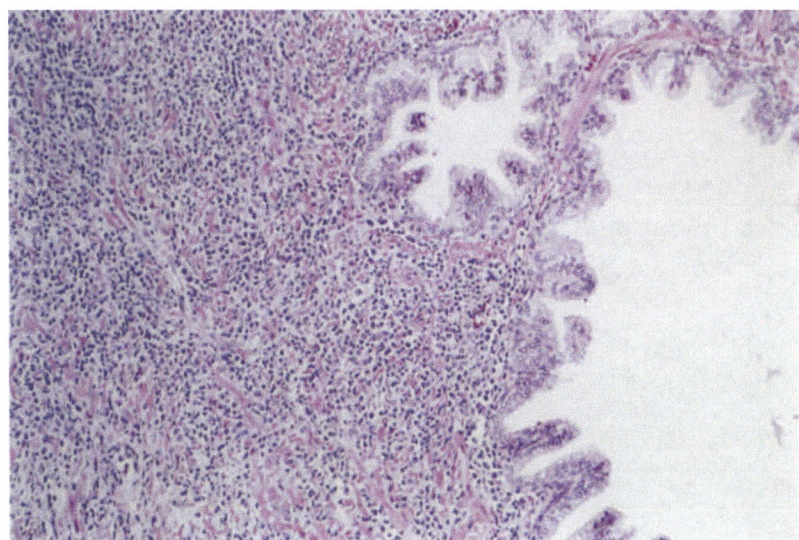

Fig. 85. Lymphoma

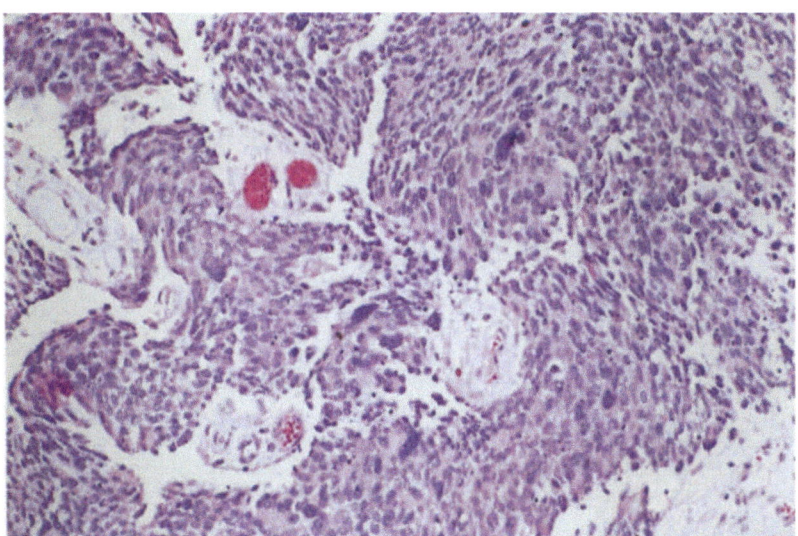

Fig. 86. Cautery artefact

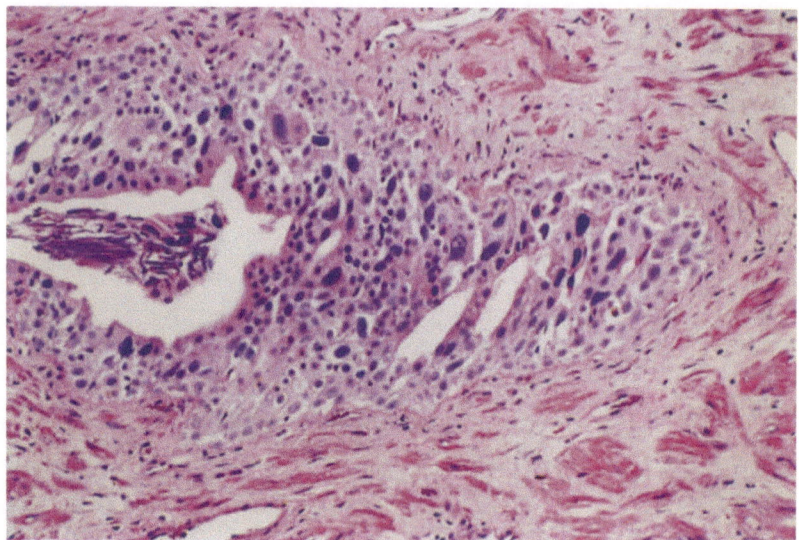

Fig. 87. Radiation effect, benign prostate

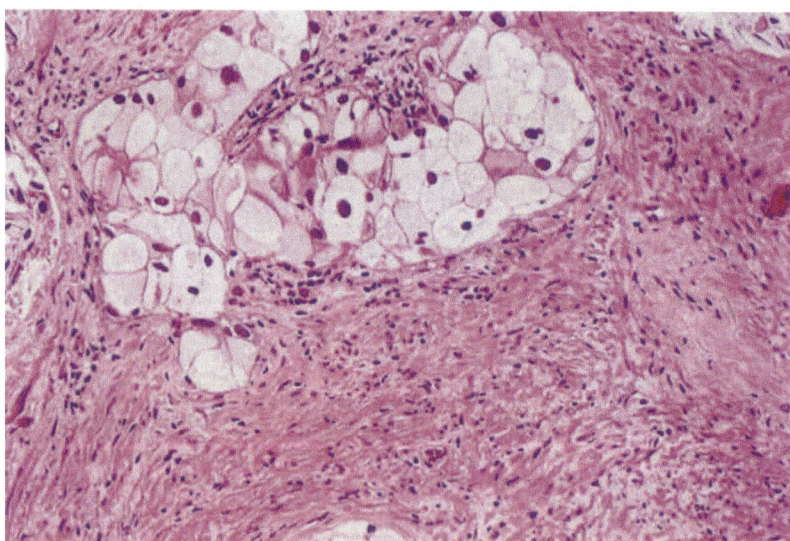

Fig. 88. Adenocarcinoma with radiation effect

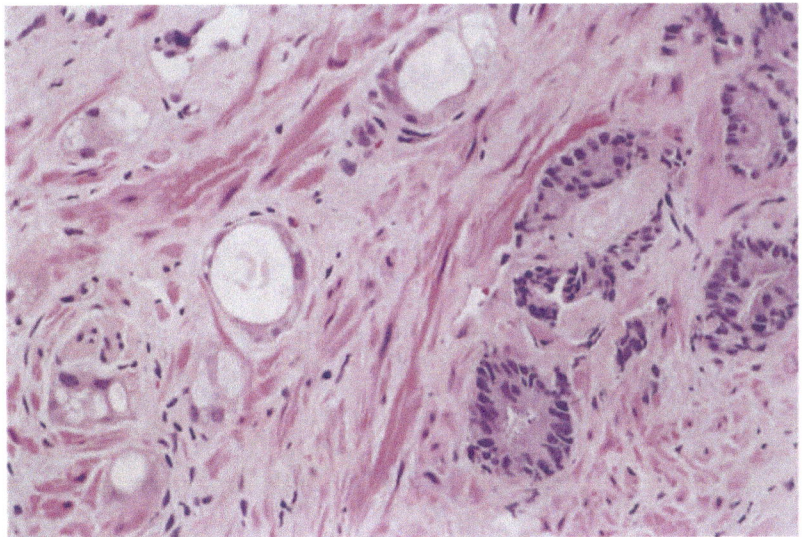

Fig. 89. Adenocarcinoma with and without radiation effect

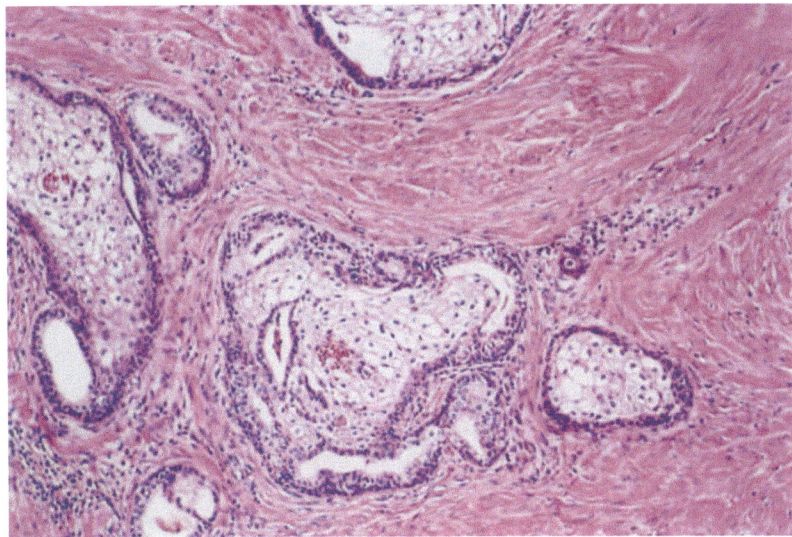

Fig. 90. Estrogen-induced squamous metaplasia

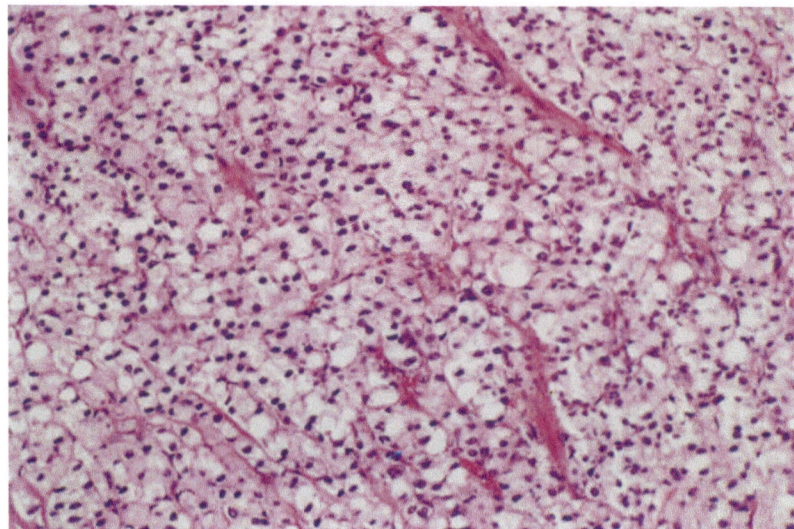

Fig. 91. Adenocarcinoma with estrogen effect

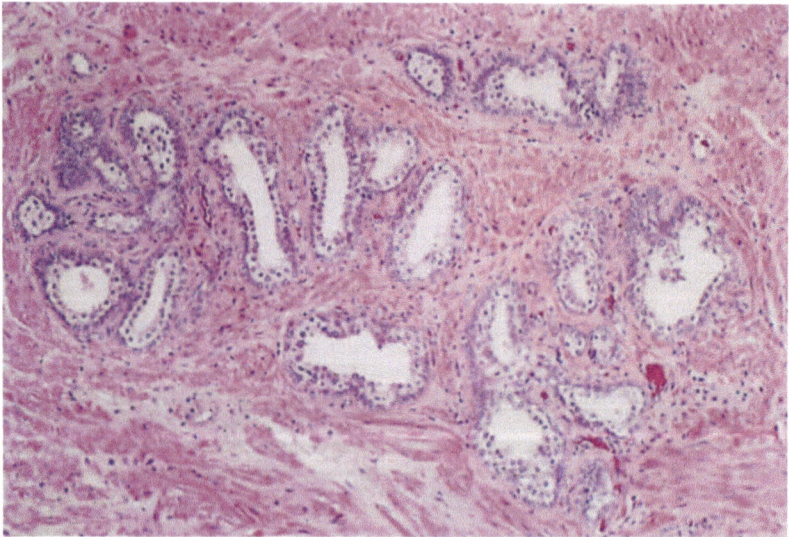

Fig. 92. Antiandrogen effect, benign prostate

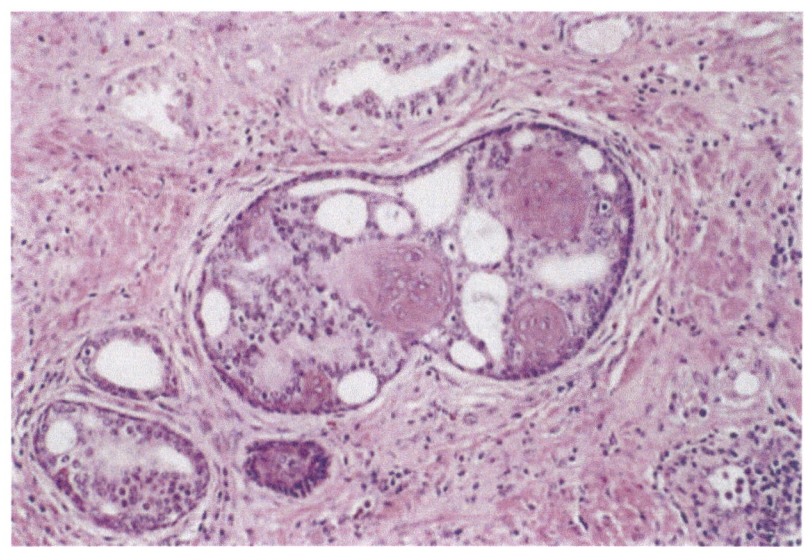

Fig. 93. Antiandrogen effect, benign gland (centre)

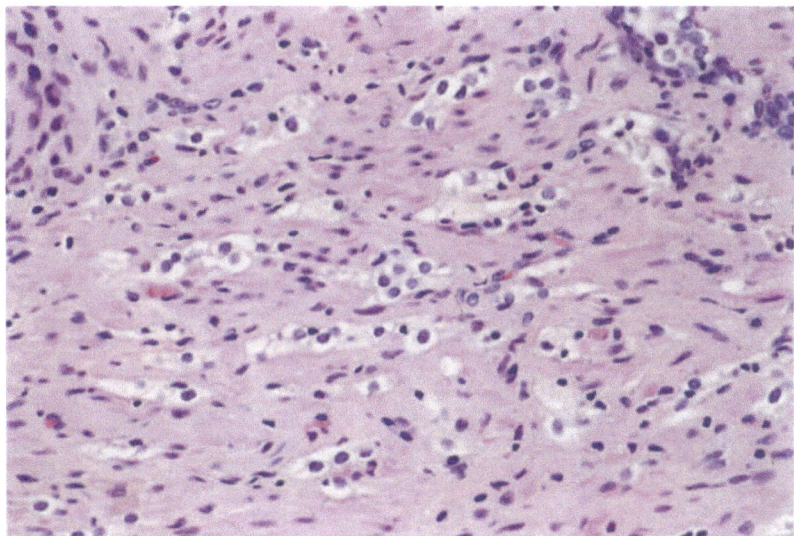

Fig. 94. Adenocarcinoma with antiandrogen effect

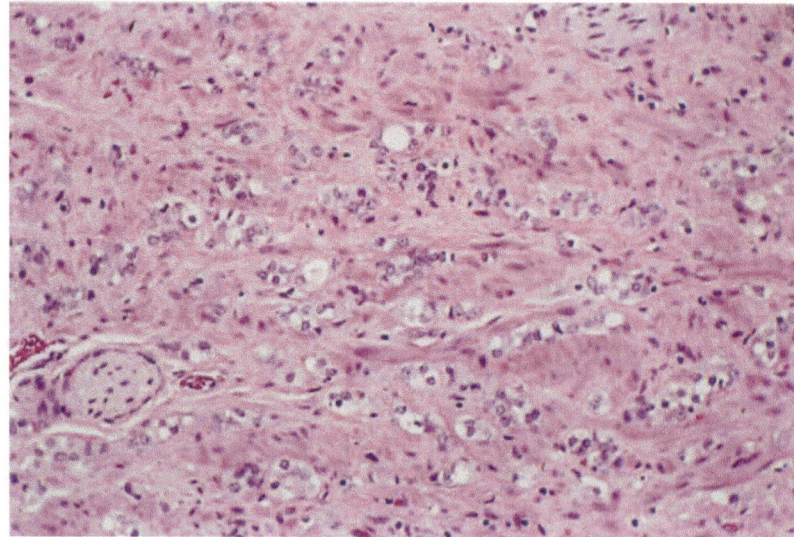

Fig. 95. Adenocarcinoma with antiandrogen effect

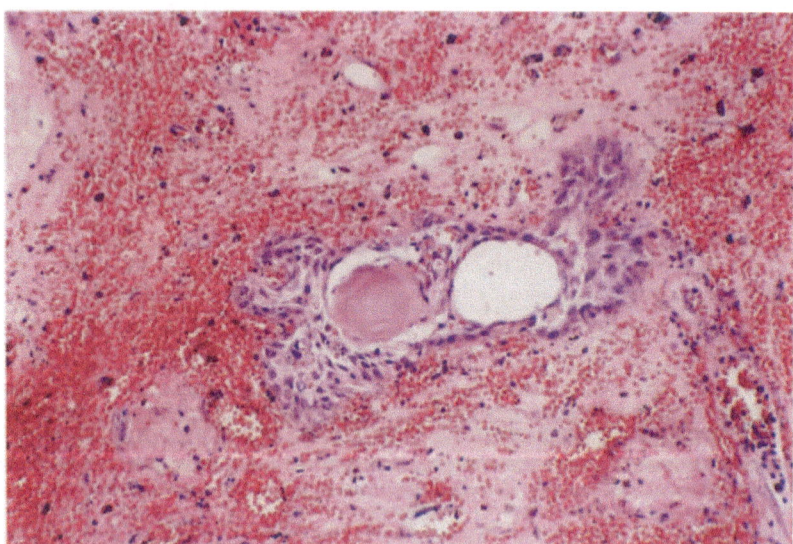

Fig. 96. Infarction

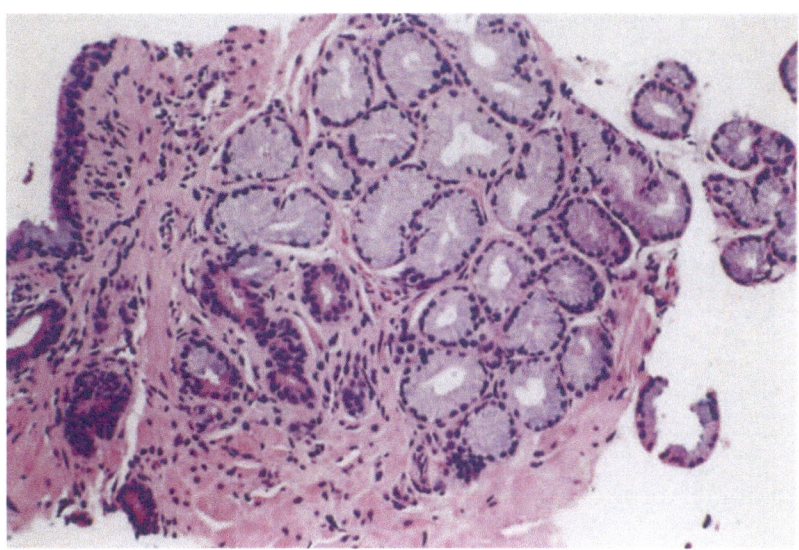

Fig. 97. Mucinous metaplasia

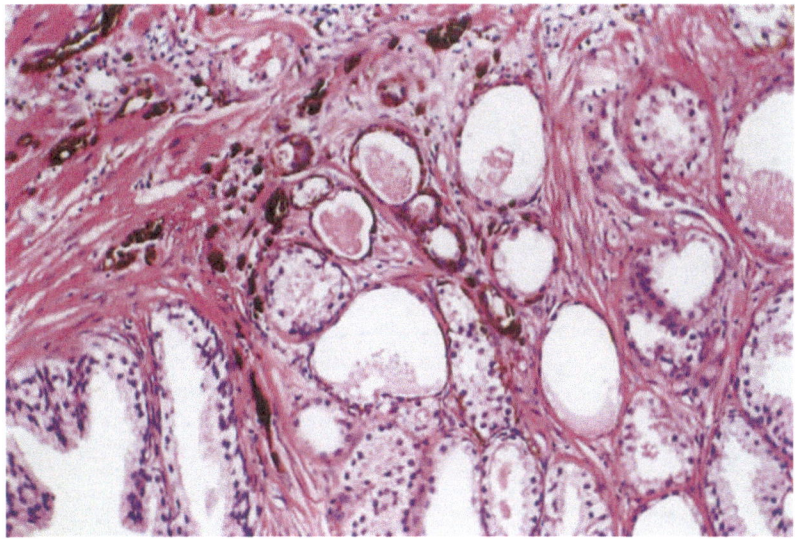

Fig. 98. Melanosis

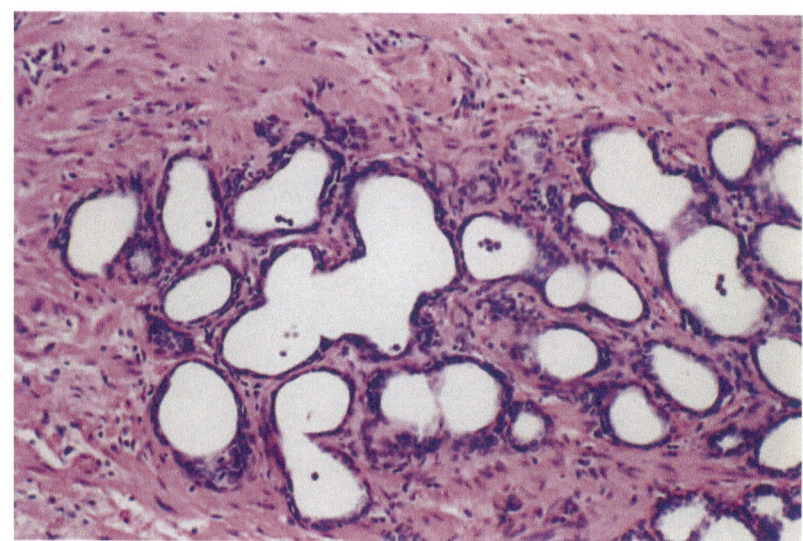

Fig. 99. Atrophy

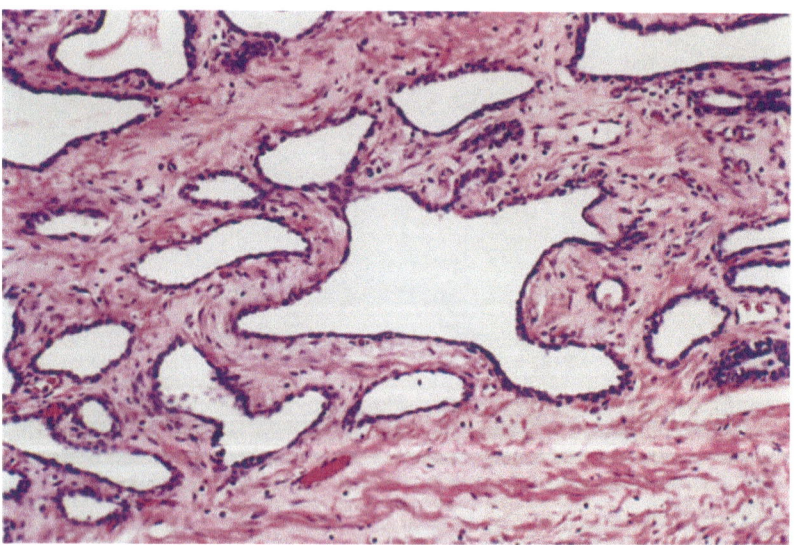

Fig. 100. Atrophy

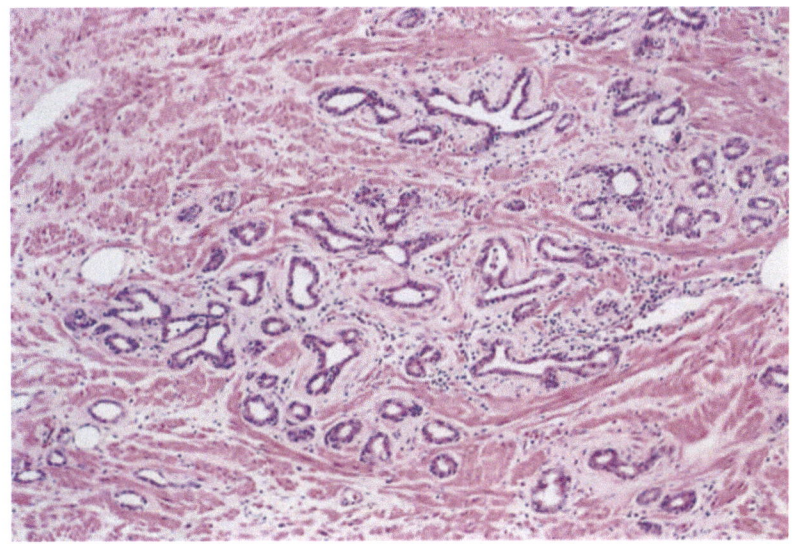

Fig. 101. Atrophy

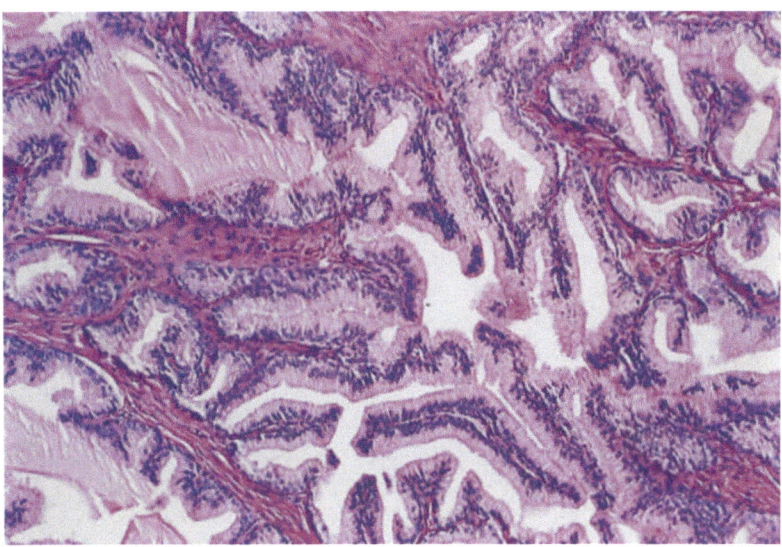

Fig. 102. Hyperplasia

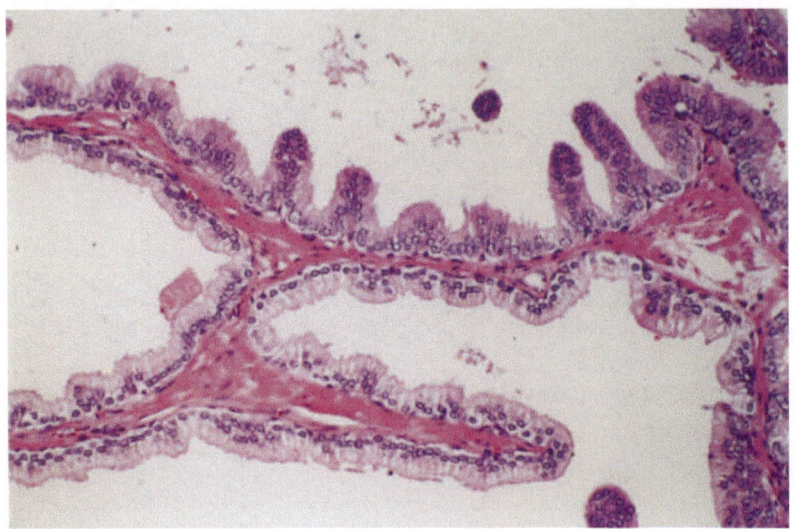

Fig. 103. Atypical hyperplasia

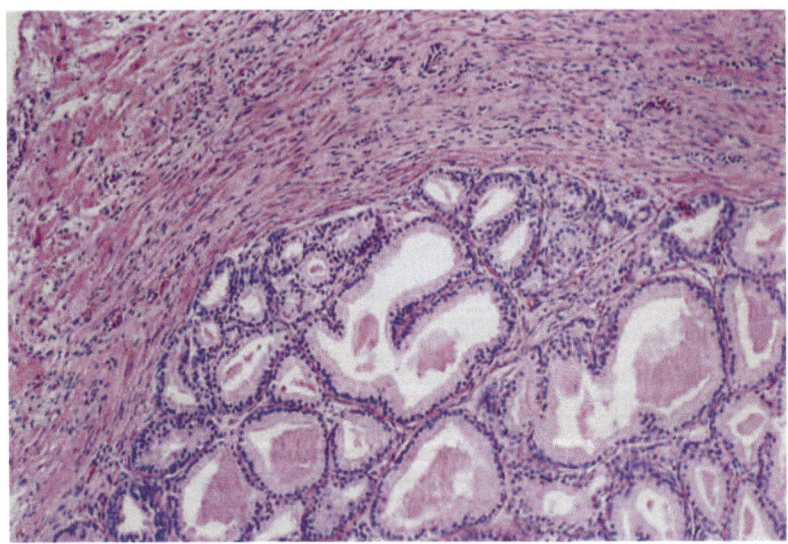

Fig. 104. Microacinar hyperplasia

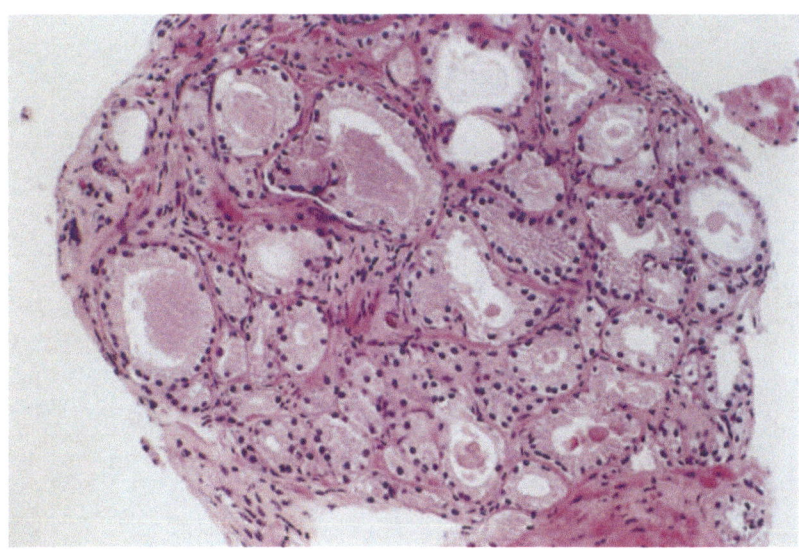

Fig. 105. Microacinar hyperplasia

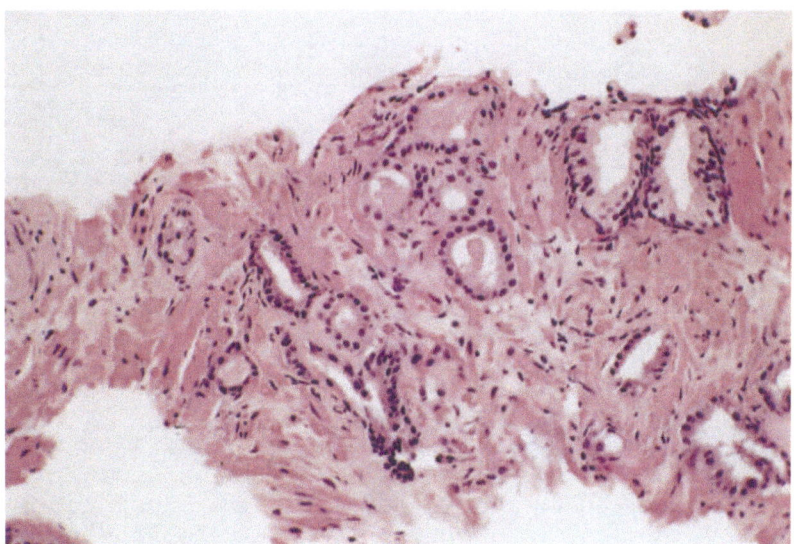

Fig. 106. Atypical glands

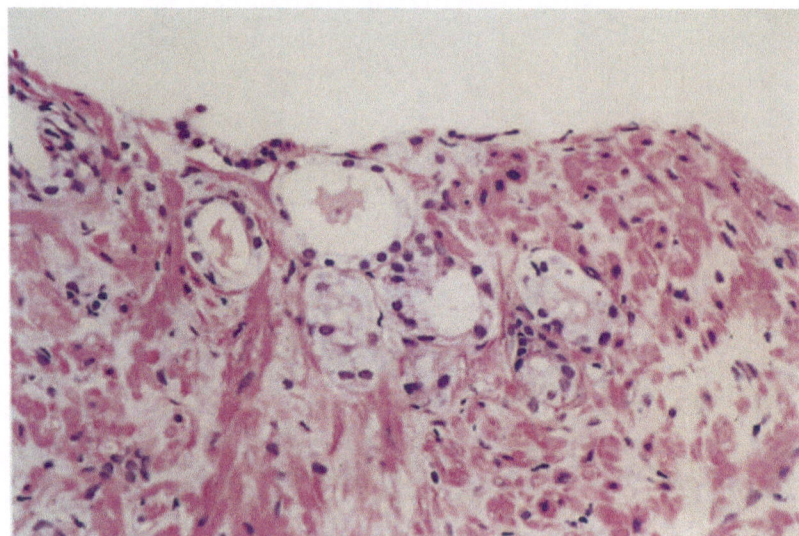

Fig. 107. Atypical glands, probably benign

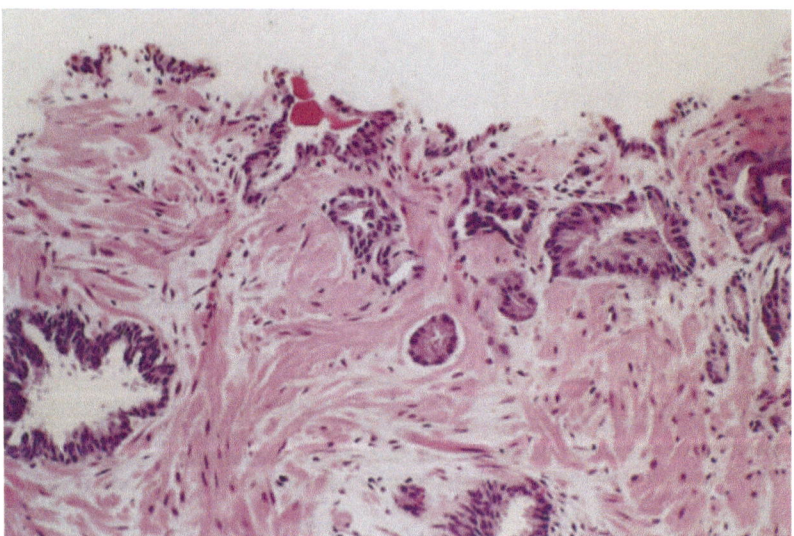

Fig. 108. Atypical glands, probably carcinoma

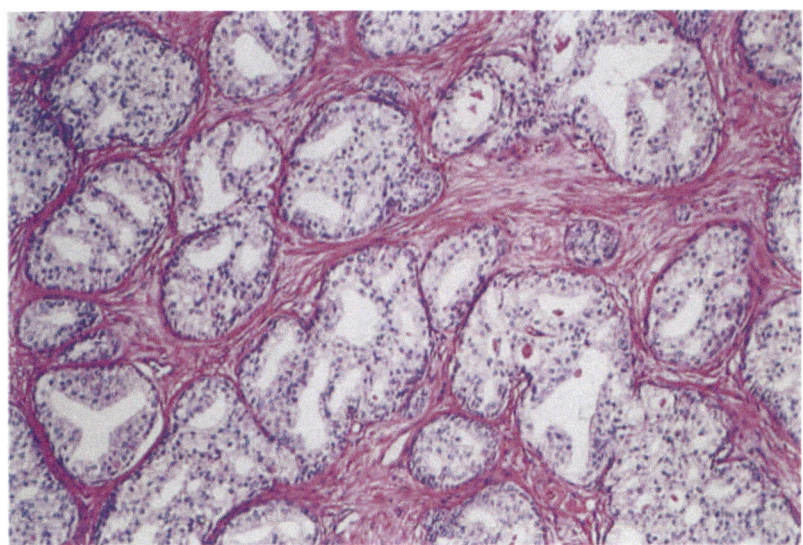

Fig. 109. Cribriform hyperplasia

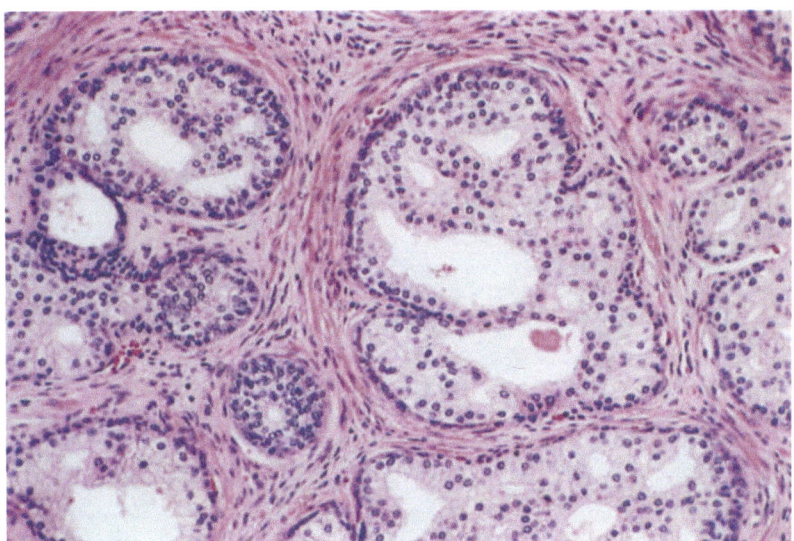

Fig. 110. Cribriform hyperplasia

92

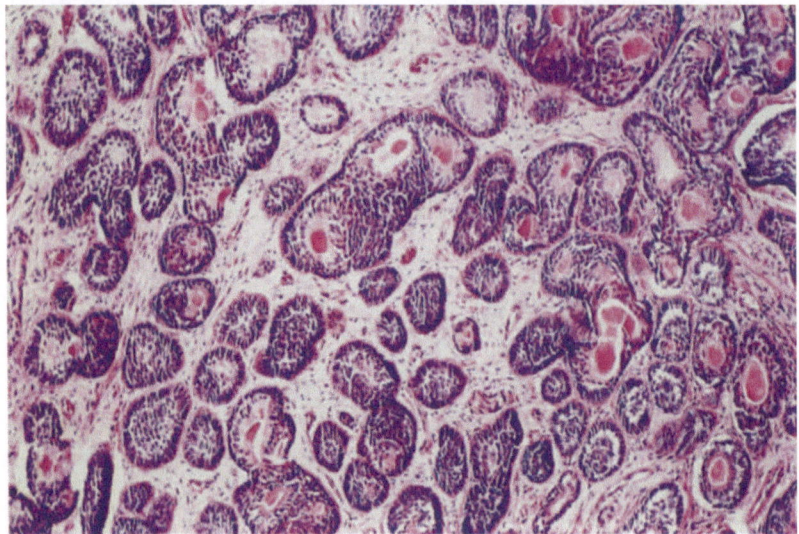

Fig. 111. Basal cell hyperplasia

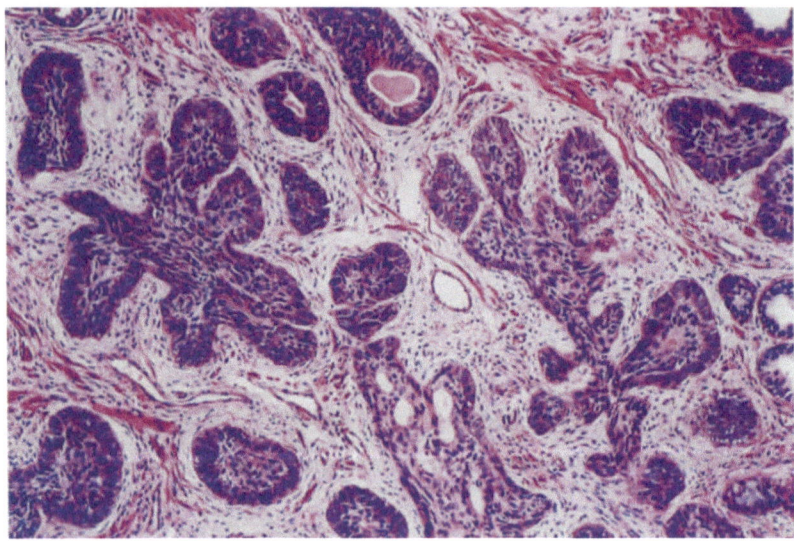

Fig. 112. Basal cell hyperplasia

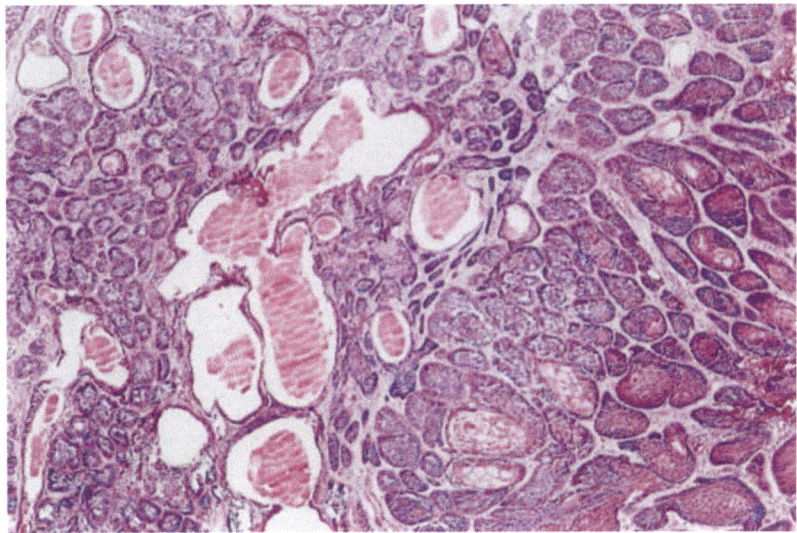

Fig. 113. Basal cell hyperplasia with squamous differentiation

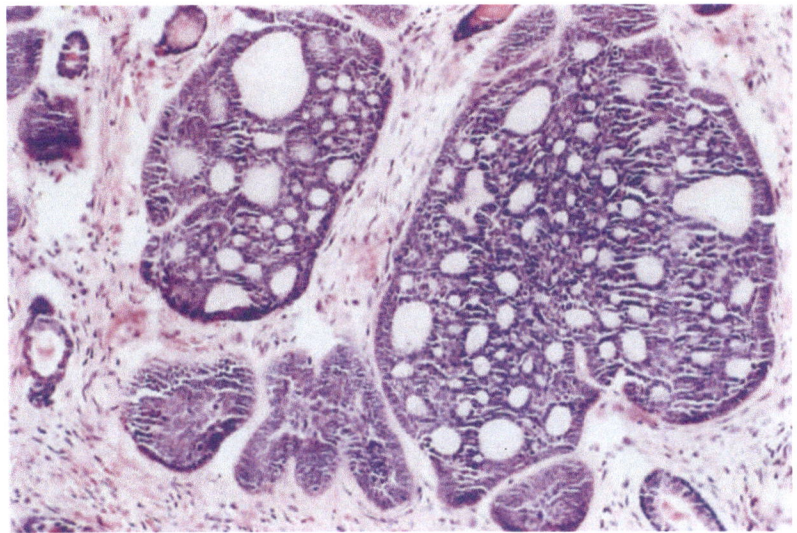

Fig. 114. Basal cell hyperplasia, adenoid cystic pattern

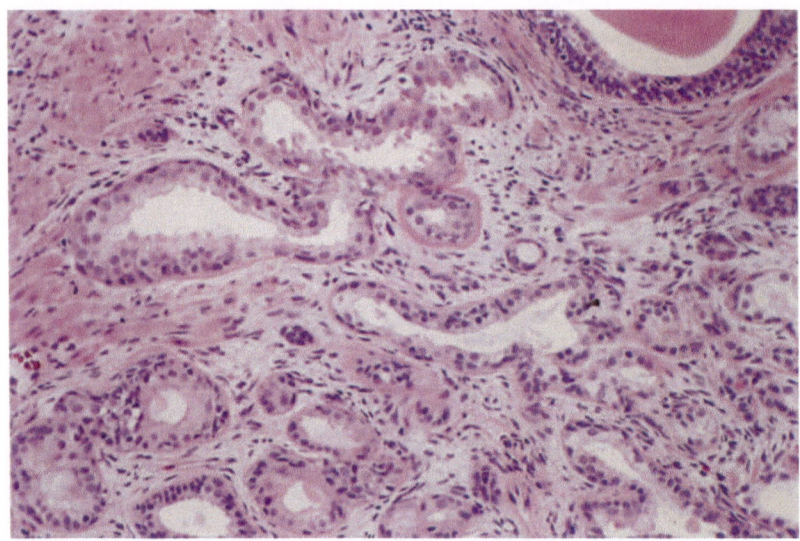

Fig. 115. Sclerosing adenosis

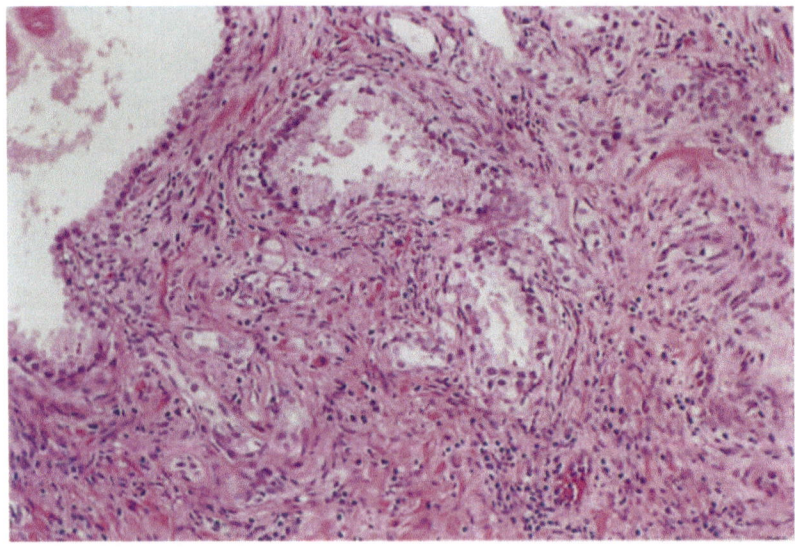

Fig. 116. Sclerosing adenosis

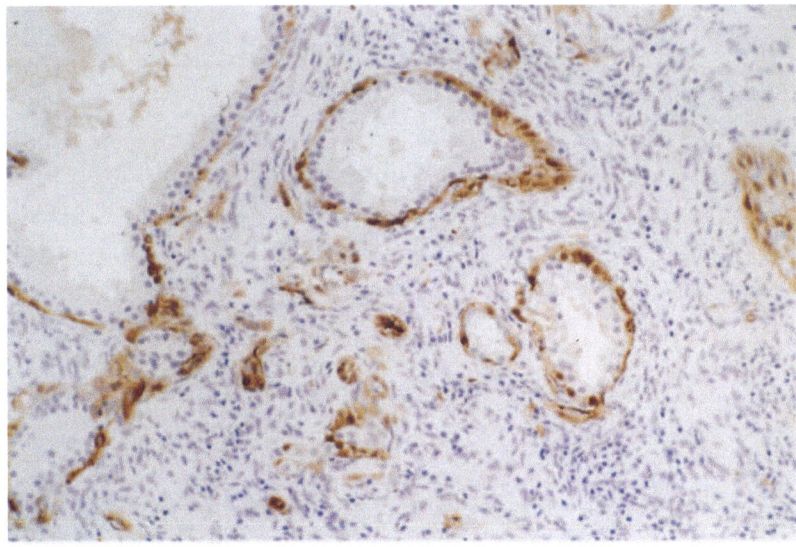

Fig. 117. Sclerosing adenosis anti-S100 highlights myoepithelial cells. Same field as Fig. 116

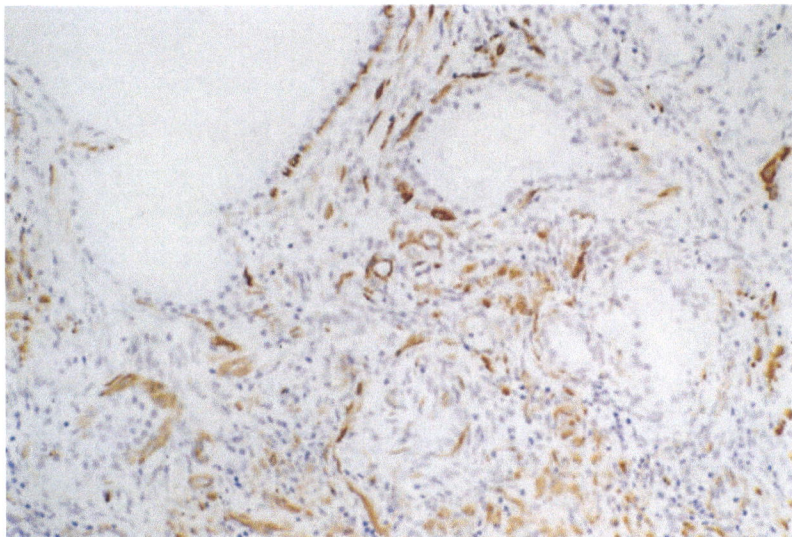

Fig. 118. Sclerosing adenosis anti-actin. Same field as Fig. 116

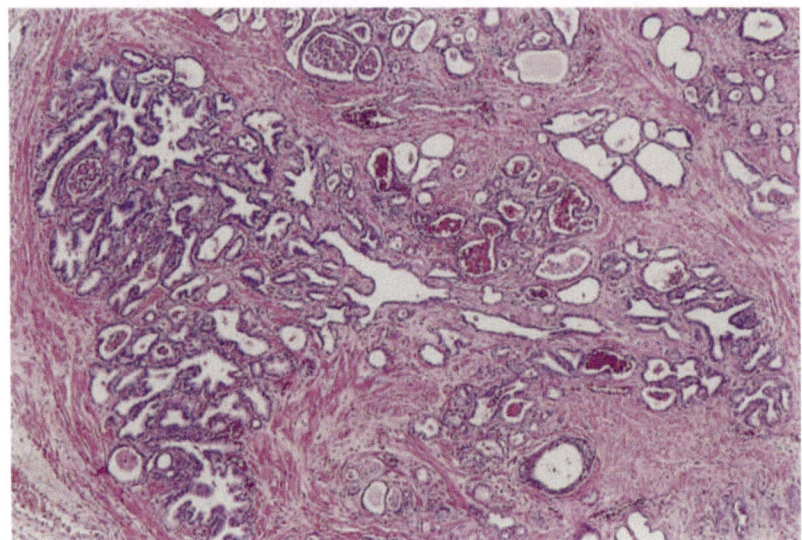

Fig. 119. Postatrophic hyperplasia

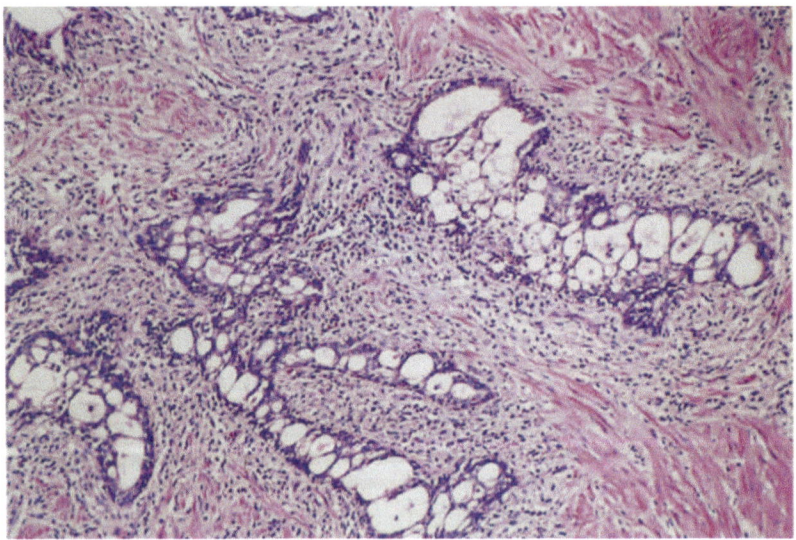

Fig. 120. Reactive epithelial hyperplasia secondary to chronic prostatitis

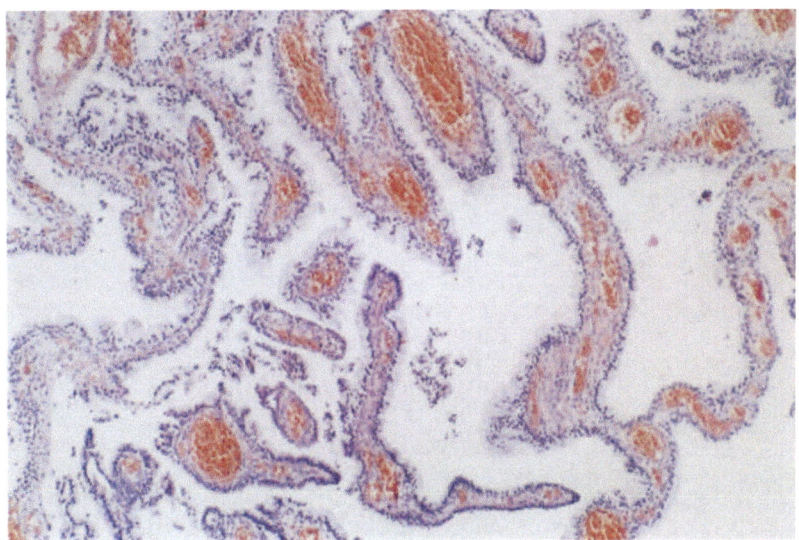

Fig. 121. Papillary hyperplasia

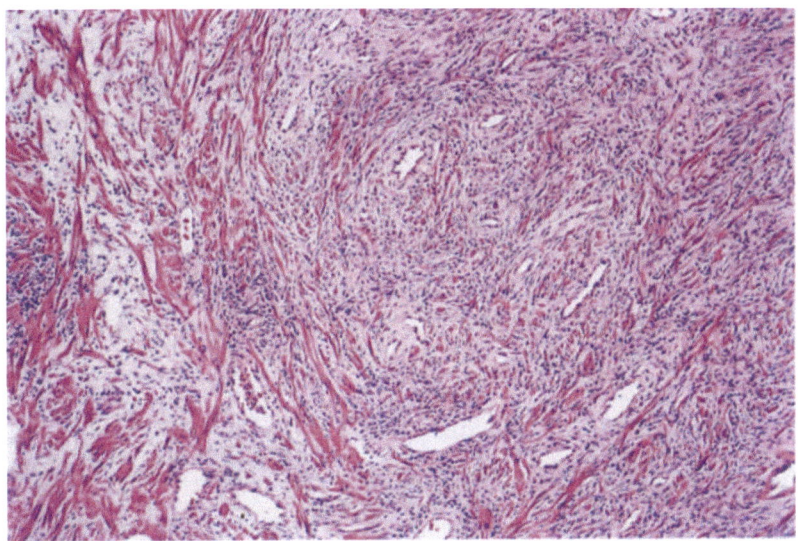

Fig. 122. Prostatic stromal hyperplasia

98

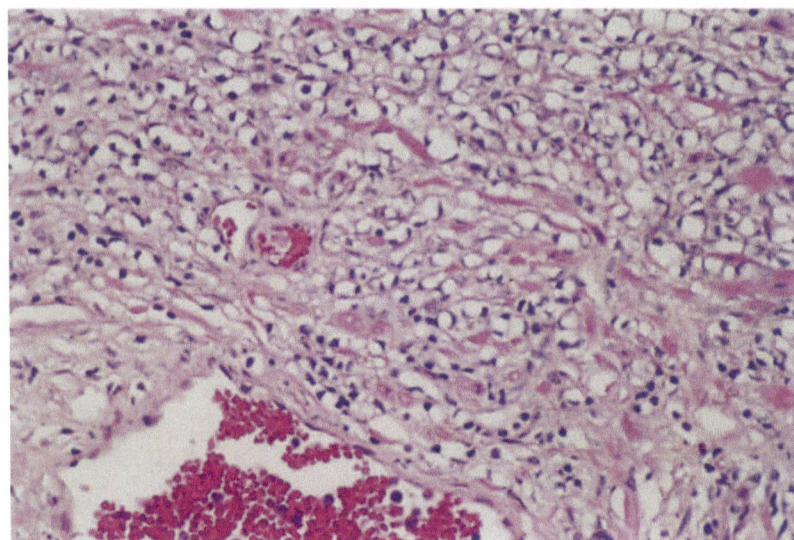

Fig. 123. Chronic prostatitis with lymphocytes showing signet ring artefact

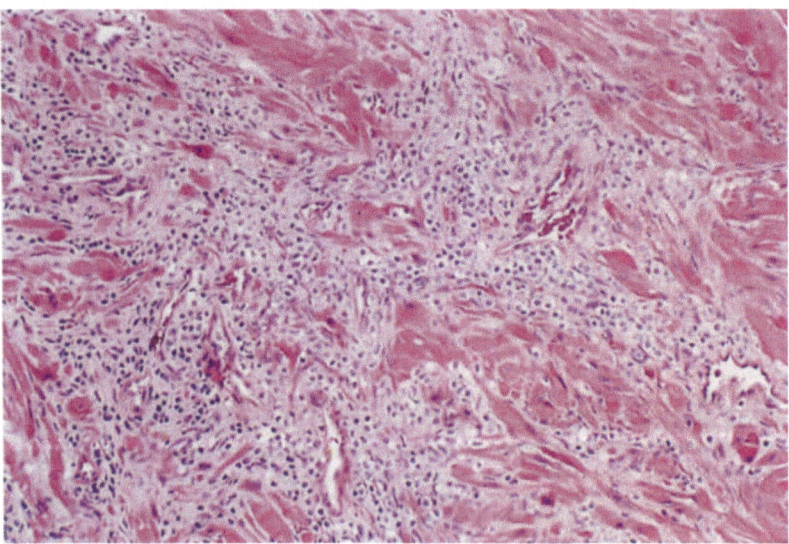

Fig. 124. Chronic prostatitis with lymphocytes showing peripheral halos

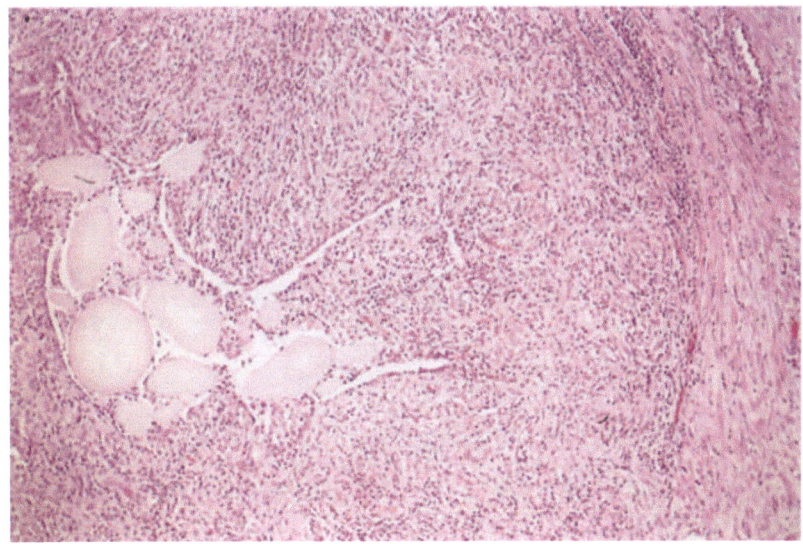

Fig. 125. Nonspecific granulomatous prostatitis

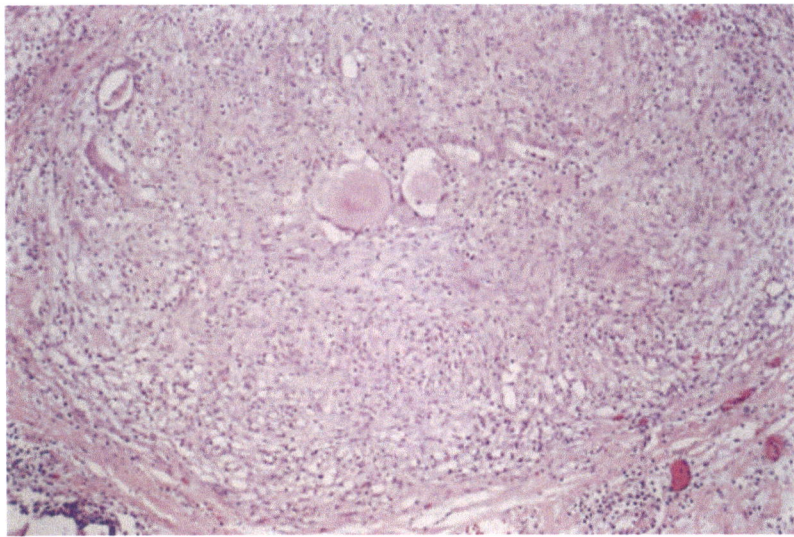

Fig. 126. Nonspecific granulomatous prostatitis

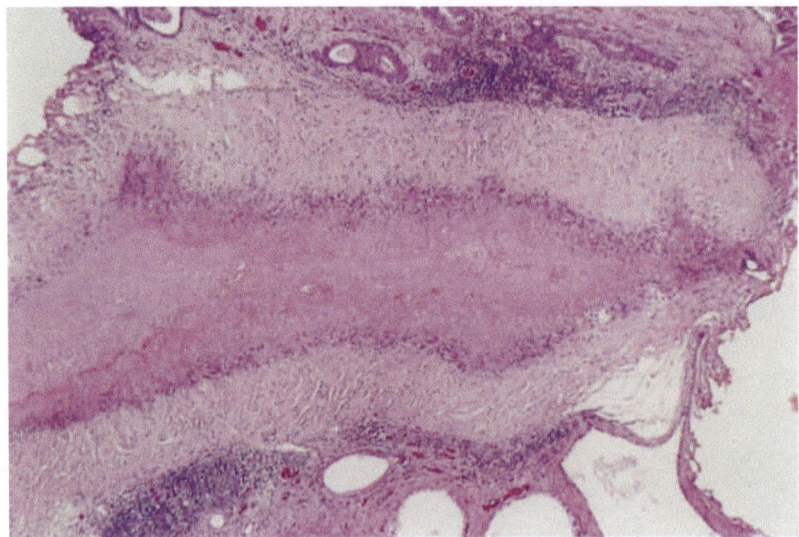

Fig. 127. Post TUR granuloma

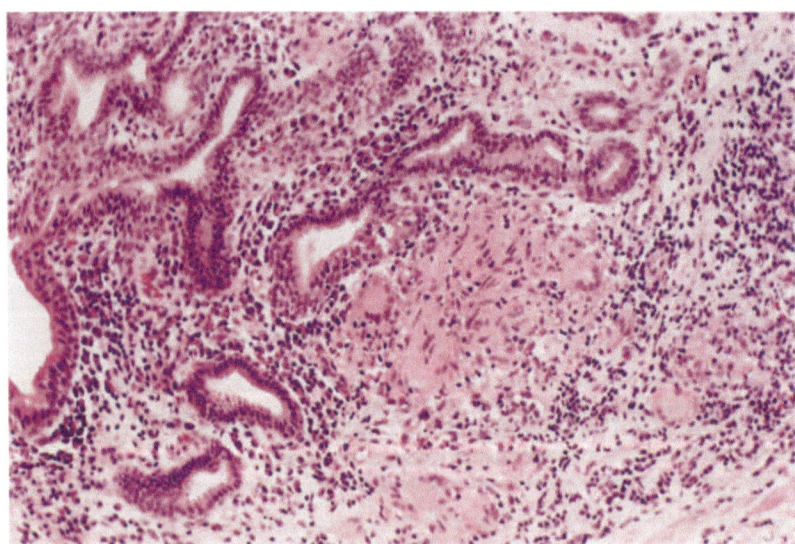

Fig. 128. Epithelioid granuloma following BCG treatment

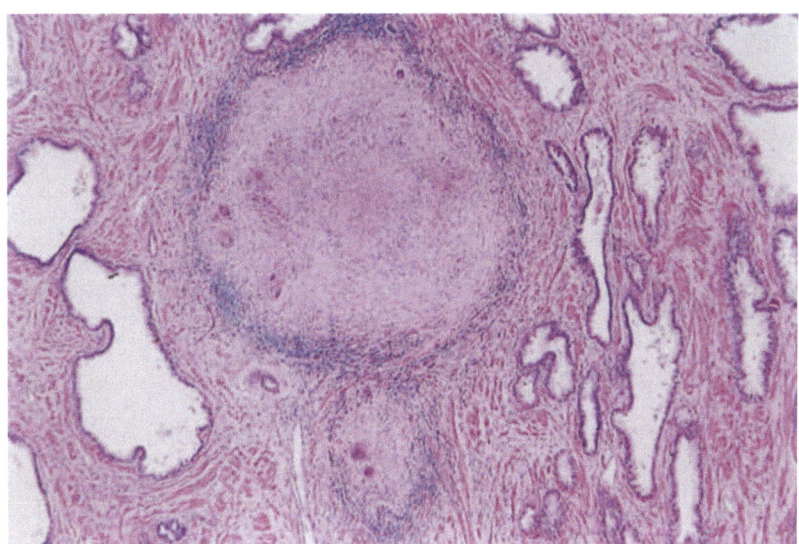

Fig. 129. Granuloma due to latent cryptococcus

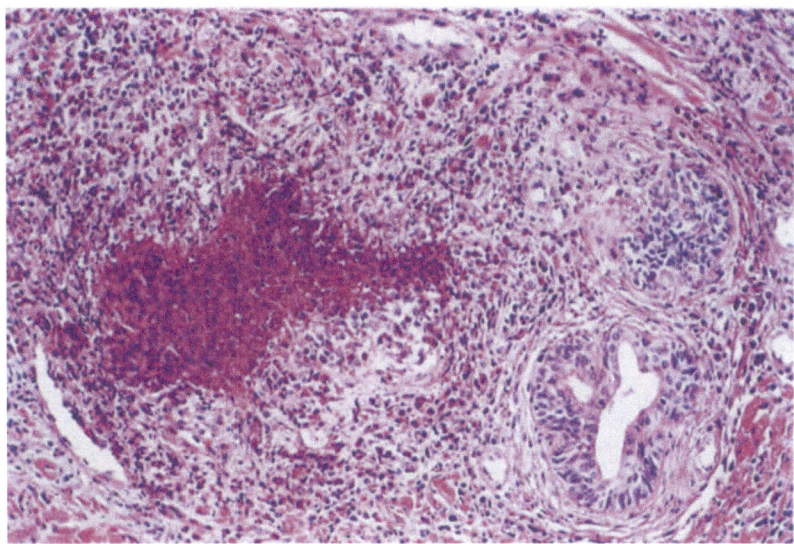

Fig. 130. Allergic granuloma

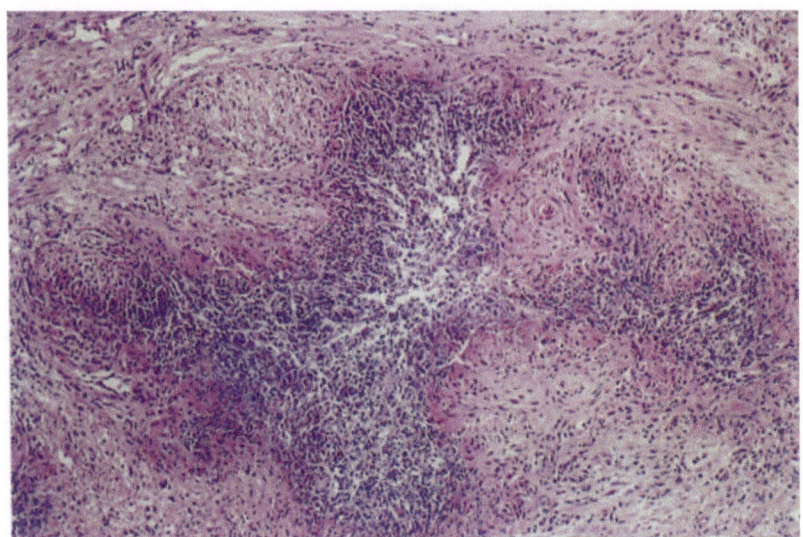

Fig. 131. Wegener's granulomatosis

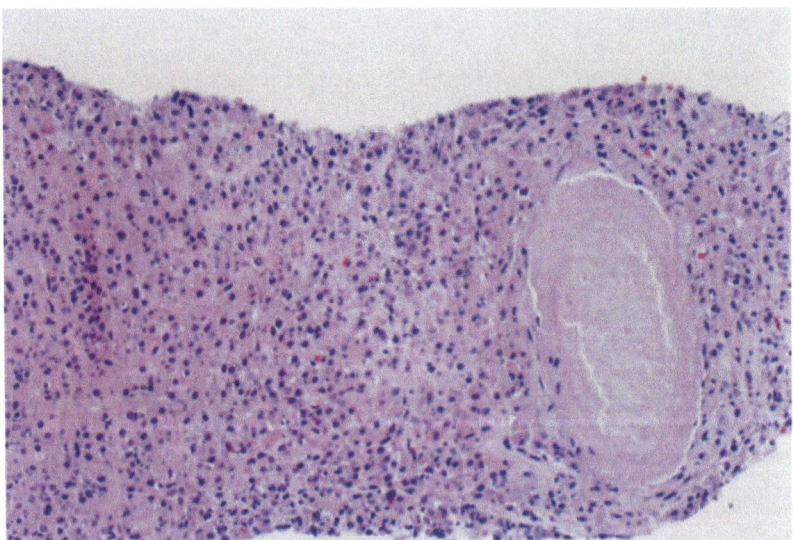

Fig. 132. Malakoplakia

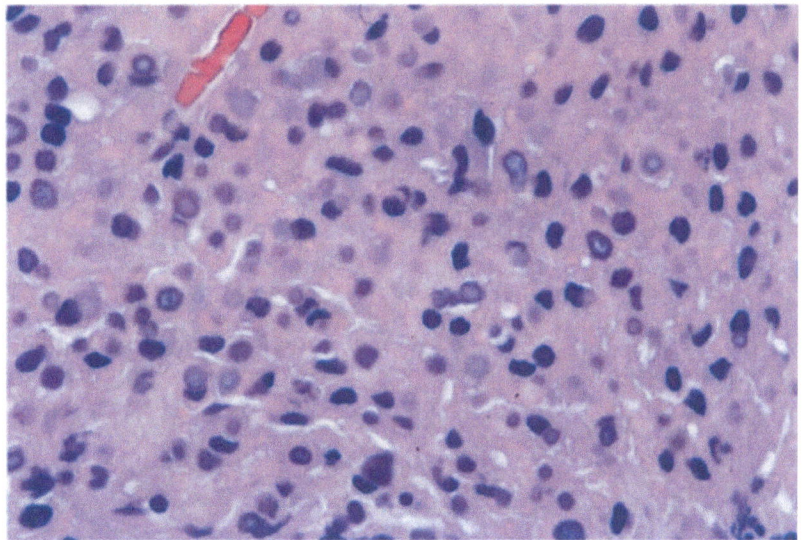

Fig. 133. Malakoplakia. Same case as Fig. 132

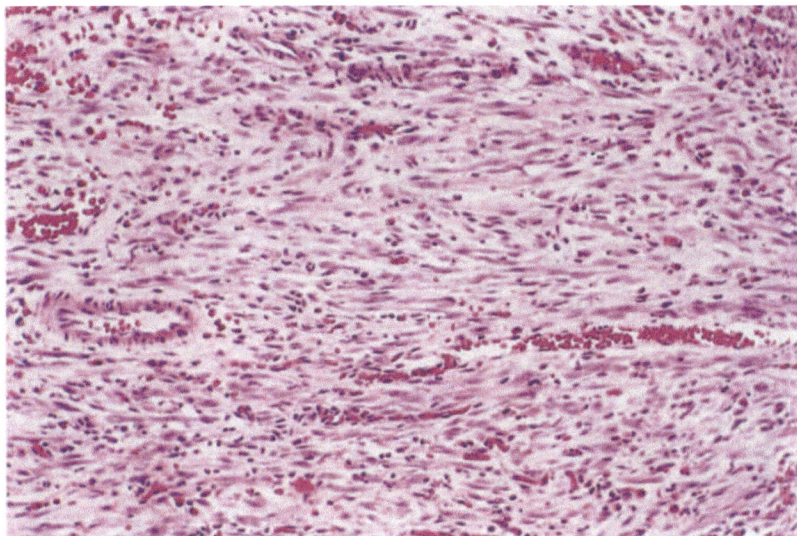

Fig. 134. Postoperative spindle cell nodule

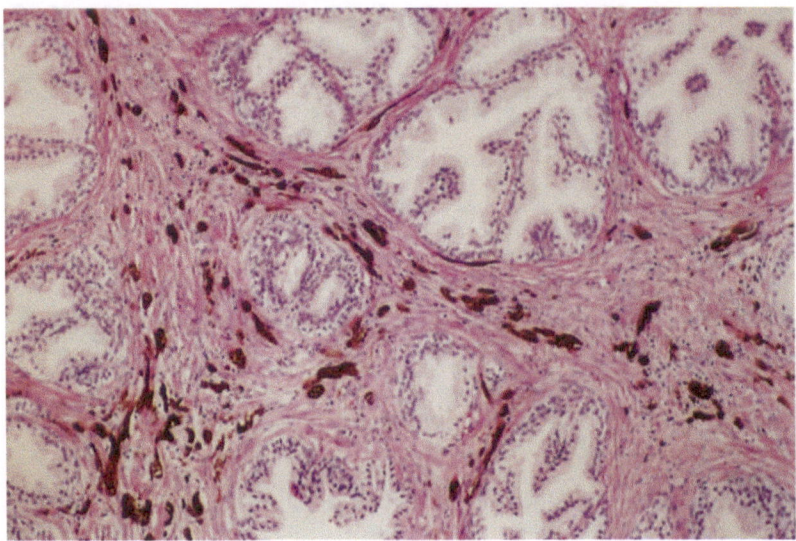

Fig. 135. Naevus

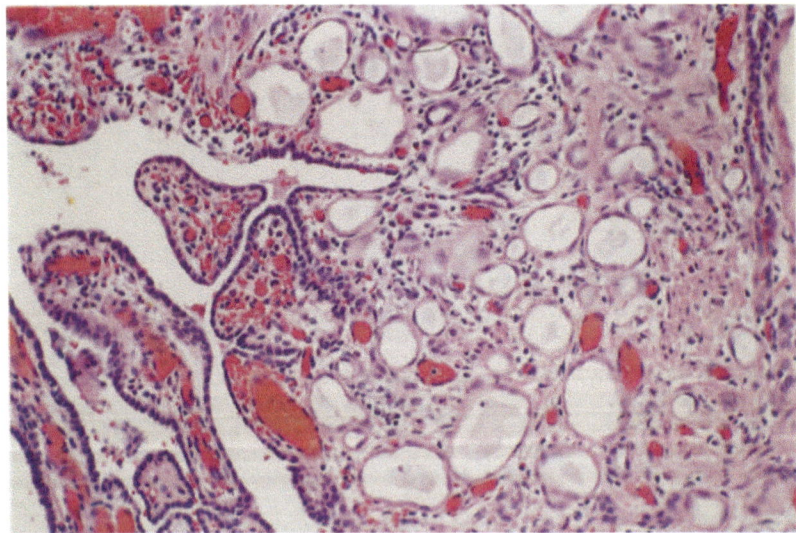

Fig. 136. Nephrogenic adenoma

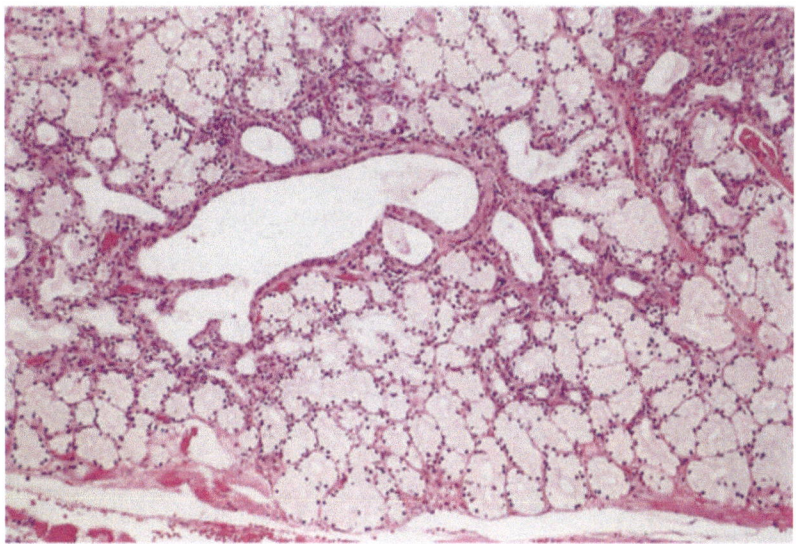

Fig. 137. Cowper glands

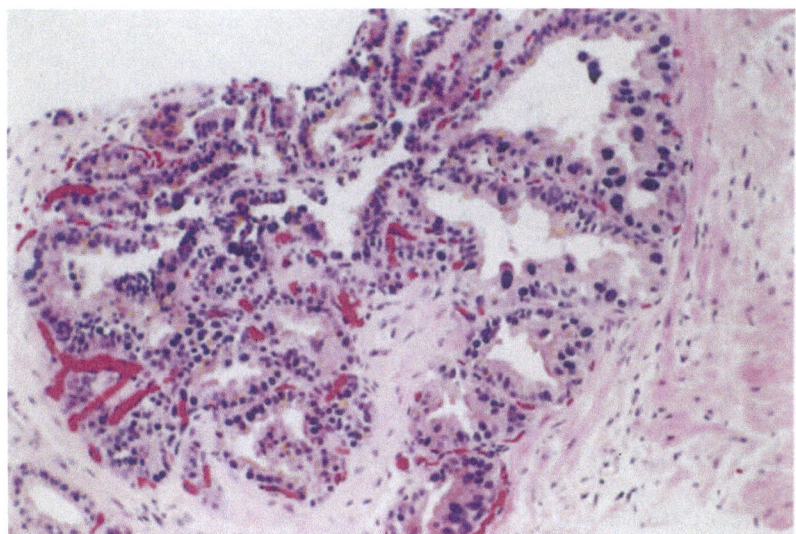

Fig. 138. Seminal vesicle with involutional change

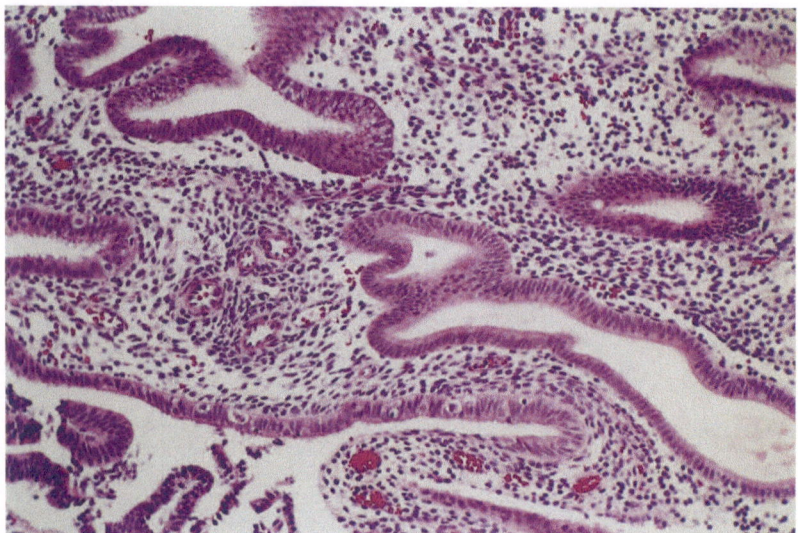

Fig. 139. Endometriosis

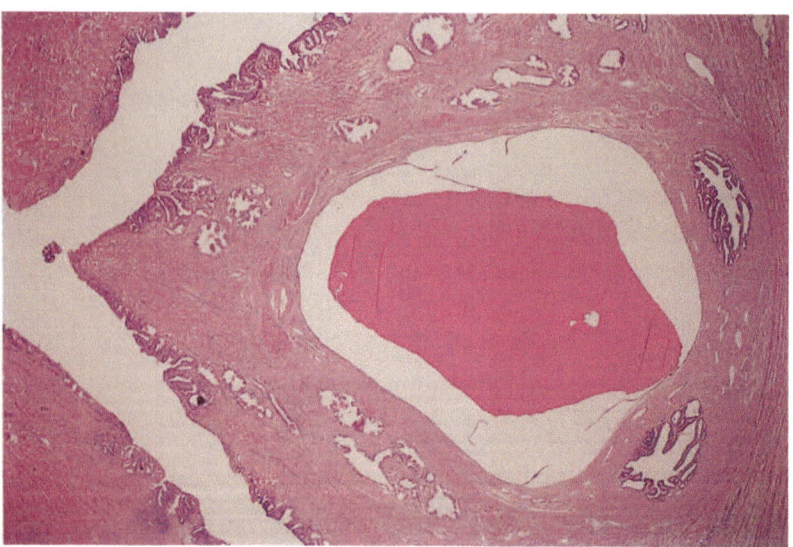

Fig. 140. Cyst of utricle

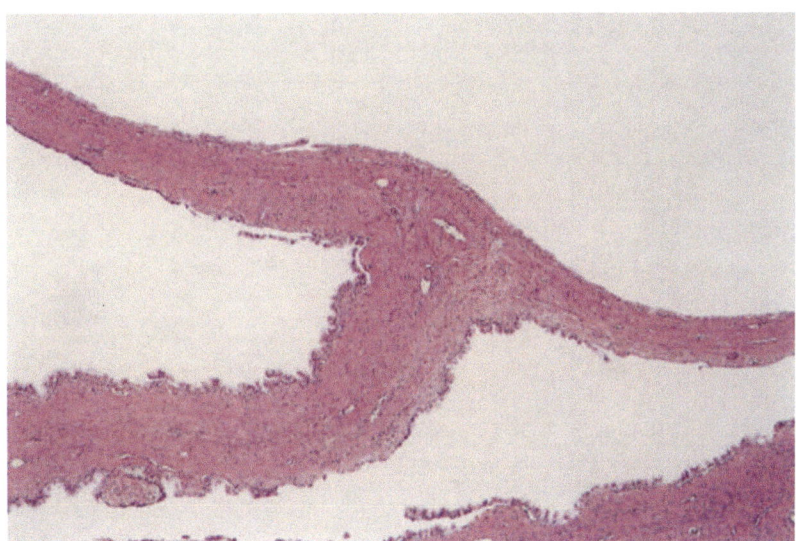

Fig. 141. Megacystic prostate

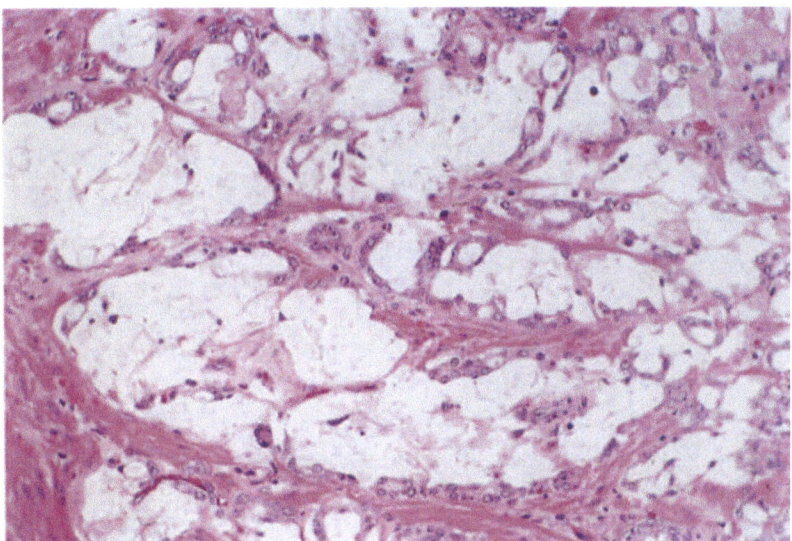

Fig. 142. Cystic change due to antiandrogen therapy

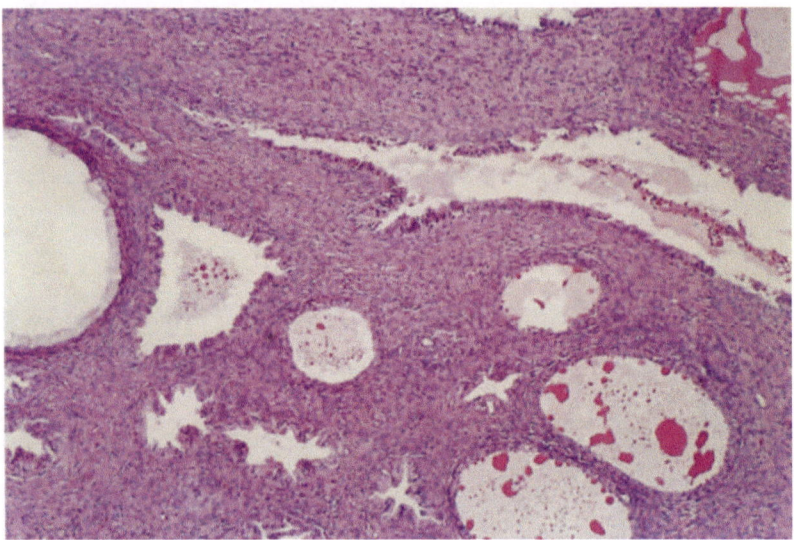

Fig. 143. Cystadenofibroma, seminal vesicle

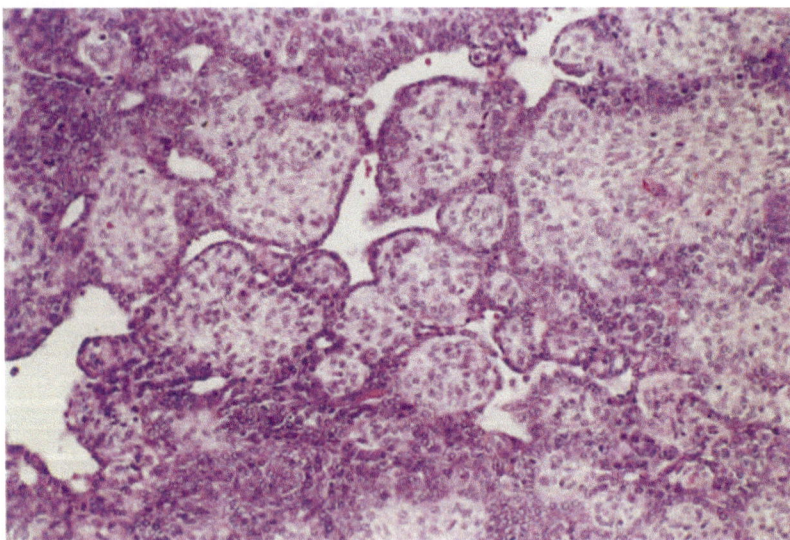

Fig. 144. Cystadenofibroma, seminal vesicle with polypoid features

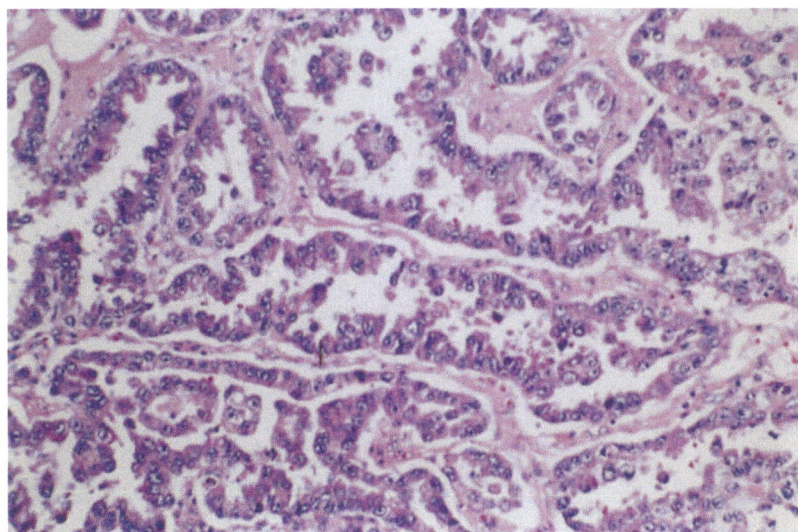

Fig. 145. Adenocarcinoma, seminal vesicle

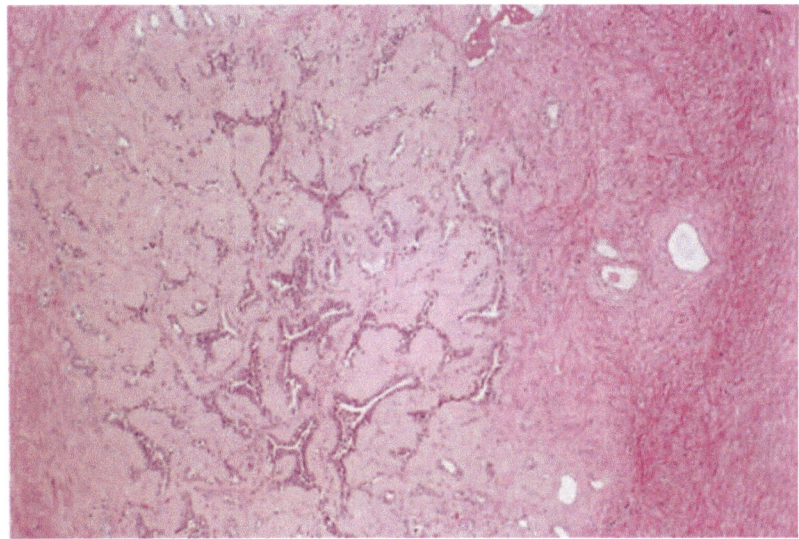

Fig. 146. Amyloidosis of seminal vesicle

Subject Index